Nursing Workforce Development

Strategic State Initiatives

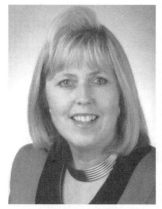

Brenda Lewis Cleary, PhD, RN, FAAN, received a BSN and an MSN from Indiana University and a doctorate in nursing from the University of Texas at Austin. Until July of 1994, Dr. Cleary was Regional Dean and Professor at Texas Tech University Health Sciences Center School of Nursing, where she received the Excellence in Teaching Award and the President's Academic Achievement Award. She currently holds the position of Executive Director of the North Carolina Center for Nursing, a state-funded agency committed to ensuring sufficient nursing resources to meet the health care needs of the citizens of North Carolina. Dr. Cleary served as project director for an initiative funded by the Robert Wood Johnson Foundation (Colleagues in Caring), the NC Nurse Workforce Planning Model, and she currently serves as a Magnet appraiser for the American Nurses Credentialing Center. She also serves on the North Carolina Institute of Medicine, a gubernatorial appointment, and is a Sigma Theta Tau Virginia Henderson fellow and a fellow in the American Academy of Nursing. She also was selected as a Robert Wood Johnson Executive Nurse Fellow, 2002 cohort.

Dr. Cleary has published numerous articles and book chapters related to the nursing workforce and nursing leadership, as well as an award-winning book on conducting research in long term-care settings.

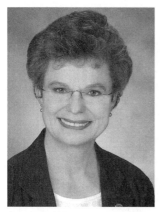

Rebecca B. Rice, EdD, RN, MPH, is currently employed as a Legislative Consultant at Macaulay & Burtch, PC, in Richmond, Virginia. In that position, she lobbies for the Commonwealth Midwives Alliance and the Virginia Dietetics Association and assists other lobbyists with advocacy work. She also codirects the Virginia Quality Healthcare Network.

Prior to moving to Richmond in July 2003, Dr. Rice served as Deputy Director of Colleagues in Caring: Regional Collaboratives for Nursing Work Force Development, a national program funded by the Robert Wood Johnson Foundation. She holds bachelor's and master's degrees in nursing from the University of Pennsylvania, a master's of public health from Virginia Commonwealth University, and a doctorate in higher education from the College of William & Mary in Virginia.

Dr. Rice is a past-president of the Virginia Nurses Association. Currently, she chairs the Legislative Coalition of Virginia Nurses and is Vice President of the Virginia Partnership for Nursing. She is a member of Sigma Theta Tau International, the Virginia Public Health Association, the National and Virginia Leagues for Nursing, the American Organization of Nurse Executives, and the American Diabetes Association. She is a contributing editor for the *American Journal of Nursing* and serves on the editorial review panel for the *Journal of Nursing Education* and the D.C. metro advisory board for *Nursing Spectrum.*

Nursing Workforce Development

Strategic State Initiatives

Brenda Cleary, PhD, RN, FAAN   **Rebecca Rice,** EdD, RN

Editors

 Springer Publishing Company

Springer Publishing Company, Inc.
11 West 42nd Street
New York, NY 10036

Acquisitions Editor: Ruth Chasek
Production Editor: Jeanne Libby
Cover design by Joanne Honigman

05 06 07 08 09 / 5 4 3 2 1

Library of Congress Cataloging-in-Publication Data

Cleary, Brenda Lewis.
  Nursing workforce development : strategic state initiatives / Brenda Cleary, Rebecca Rice.
       p. ; cm.
  Includes bibliographical references and index.
  ISBN 0-8261-2645-6
  1. Nurses—Supply and demand—United States. 2. Nurses—Supply and demand—United States—Planning. I. Rice, Rebecca, RN. II. Title.
  [DNLM: 1. Nurses—supply & distribution—United States.
2. Nursing—manpower—United States. 3. Cooperative Behavior—United States. 4. Regional Health Planning—organization & adminis-tration—United States.   WY 21 C623n 2005]
  RT86.73.C54 2005
  331.12'91362173'0973—dc22
                                                                    2004030101

Printed in the United States of America by Sheridan Books.

Contents

Contributors

James W. Bevill, Jr., RN, MSN
Associate Director for
  Recruitment and Retention
NC Center for Nursing
Raleigh, North Carolina

Michael Bleich, PhD, RN, CNAA-BC
Associate Dean, Clinical and
  Community Affairs
Executive Director/COO,
  KU HealthPartners, Inc.
The University of Kansas School
  of Nursing
Kansas City, Kansas

Susan A. Boyer, MEd, RN
Director, Vermont Nurse
  Internship Project
Perkinsville, Vermont

Mary Lou Brunell, MSN, RN
Executive Director
Florida Center for Nursing
Orlando, Florida

Edna Cadmus, PhD, RN, CNAA
Senior Vice President, Patient
  Care Services
Englewood Hospital and Medical
  Center
Englewood, New Jersey

Joyce Clifford, PhD, RN, FAAN
Executive Director
The Institute for Nursing
  Healthcare Leadership
Boston, Massachusetts

Karen S. Cox, PhD, RN
Senior Vice President, Patient
  Care Services
Children's Mercy Hospital and
  Clinics
Kansas City, Missouri

Geri Dickson, PhD, RN
Executive Director
The New Jersey Collaborating
  Center for Nursing Workforce
  Development
Rutgers College of Nursing
Newark, New Jersey

Ann Duncan, MPH, RN
Executive Director
Tennessee Center for Nursing, Inc.
Nashville, Tennessee

Jill Fuller, PhD, RN
Vice President, Patient Care Services
Prairie Lakes Healthcare System
Watertown, South Dakota

Kathryn V. Hall, MS, RN
Executive Director
Maryland Nurses Association
Project Director, Maryland
  Colleagues in Caring
Baltimore, Maryland

Donna Sullivan Havens, PhD, RN, FAAN
Professor and Division Chair
The University of North Carolina
  at Chapel Hill School of Nursing
Chapel Hill, North Carolina

Marge Hegge, EdD, MS, RN
Distinguished Professor Emeritus
Coordinator, Nursing Accelerated
   Program
South Dakota State University
Sioux Falls, South Dakota

**Peggy O'Neill Hewlett, PhD, RN,
   FAAN**
Associate Dean for Research
University of Mississippi Medical
   Center School of Nursing
2500 N. State Street
Jackson, Mississippi

Kim Welch Hoover, PhD, RN
Associate Dean, Academic
   Program Development and
   Evaluation
University of Mississippi Medical
   Center School of Nursing
Jackson, Mississippi

Edith Irving, MS, RN
Chief Nursing Officer
Eastern Idaho Regional Medical
   Center
Idaho Falls, Idaho

Claudia Johnston, PhD, RN
Associate Vice President for
   Academic Affairs
Texas A&M, University—Corpus
   Christi
Corpus Christi, Texas

Linda M. Lacey, MA
Associate Director for Research
NC Center for Nursing
Raleigh, North Carolina

Susan Lacey, PhD, RN
Associate Professor of Nursing
University of Alabama
Huntsville, Alabama

**Judith Kline Leavitt, MEd, RN,
   FAAN**
Associate Professor
University of Mississippi Medical
   Center School of Nursing
Jackson, Mississippi

Ellen M. Lewis, MSN, RN, FAAN
Program Administrator, Nursing
   and Allied Health
College of Medicine
University of California, Irvine
Irvine, California

**Renatta S. Loquist, MN, RN,
   FAAN**
Former Director, South Carolina
   Colleagues in Caring
Columbia, South Carolina

Marcella M. McKay, PhD, RN
President/CEO
Mississippi Hospital Association
   Health, Research and
   Educational Foundation, Inc.
Jackson, Mississippi

**Barbara S. Mitchell, MSN, MS,
   RN, BC**
Executive Director, Nursing 2000
Indianapolis, Indiana

Eileen T. O'Grady, PhD, RN, NP
The George Washington University
Washington, D.C.

**Cynthia Armstrong Persily,
   PhD, RN**
Associate Professor and Chair-
   person, Charleston Division
Associate Dean, Academic Affairs,
   Southern Region Programs
West Virginia University School
   of Nursing
Charleston, West Virginia

Fran Roberts, PhD, RN
Dean, Grand Canyon University
Samaritan College of Nursing
(Formerly Vice President,
    Professional Services,
    Arizona Hospital and
    Healthcare Association)
Phoenix, Arizona

Karen Sechrist, PhD, RN
Principal, Berlin Sechrist
    Associates
(Formerly Project Investigator,
    California Strategic Planning
    Committee)
Irvine, California

Dennis R. Sherrod, EdD, RN
Forsyth Medical Center Endowed
    Chair of Recruitment and
    Retention
Winston-Salem State University
Winston-Salem, North Carolina

Foreword

JoEllen Koerner, RN, PhD, FAAN

The trouble with our times is that the future is not what it used to be.
—Paul Valery

B e prepared for a breathtaking inside view of a courageous and innovative group of nursing colleagues who have rewritten traditional rules and processes to launch a national change process around a nationwide nursing shortage of unprecedented proportion. Utilizing an agenda created and managed at the grassroots level along with technological networking and innovation, a national environment for nursing was co-created which was nimble, adaptable, and relevant to people in the context of their lives. This book offers a blueprint for designing such a network.

Be empowered by the wisdom and leadership demonstrated at every level of the process. The models reflected in these chapters replace familiar patterns of power and privilege, which have existed for civilizations, with flexible social networks that fostered social entrepreneurship as a dynamic and effective vehicle for change. Tools and strategies provided in these exciting chapters guide groups beyond executing a preset agenda created by an expert panel, to strategies that establish dynamic and collaborative teams which co-create and adapt agendas at the grassroots level. The solution to any problem lies within it.

Be challenged by the way that workforce development, as represented in this book, has transcended the traditional boundaries of status, role, functional affiliation and geographic location that for years have defined and controlled our work. Timely and innovative use of web-based technologies and other networking tools and resources allowed for real-time dialogue, exploration, and co-creation, as well as quick adaptation around what did not work. Book authors model boundary-less behavior as information access and decision-making authority was moved from a 'filtering outside expert' directly to the members living the issue. In real-time they would deliberately reason together about meaning and then create preferred outcomes for their own state. Context gives form and definition to the issue at hand.

Be inspired by the new relationships, individual and organizational, that strengthened their response to the national nursing shortage, along with other social issues facing local and state government today. This collaborative model helped nursing groups form partnerships with other groups and associations, rather than telling them what to do. It established coalitions with related organizations, rather than defending turf. It changed the role of leadership from controller and authority to stimulator, catalyst, and mentor. It prompted invitations for them to new tables as their wisdom and perspective became visible to others.

'Colleagues in caring' is a global framework for initiating a change process that will continue to adapt as the new world unfolds. It is the living laboratory for the committed, compassionate, collaborative, creative, and courageous. Remember, courage is the last uncrowded place, so there is room at this table for you. Read this book and join the movement toward wholeness.

Foreword

Christine Tassone Kovner, RN, PhD, FAAN

Periodic crises about the shortage of registered nurses (RNs) have been a part of nursing since before I was a student more than thirty years ago. While all of us in health care are concerned when there is a national shortage, a subset of these groups is also concerned when there are regional or local shortages. Surpluses seem to be of almost no concern. In fact those who employ RNs and even many people in government think their problems are solved when there are surpluses. Not so for the colleges and universities that educate the next generation or the would-be RNs who see and hear in the media that there are few jobs. As writers have said for so many years the goal is to smooth the cyclical curve so both shortages and surpluses are less severe.

In times of shortage Government and Foundations often intervene with what some would say is a shot gun approach by throwing money at the problem often in the form of scholarships or subsidies to educate a new generation of RNs. Government changes immigration laws to permit RNs from abroad to come and work in the U.S. The Robert Wood Johnson Foundation took a different approach by funding the Colleagues in Caring Project, which focused funds at the regional and state levels. Like politics workforce patterns are local. Rather than providing scholarships or funding efforts to recruit people into nursing programs, the Foundation focused on state and regional workforce initiatives that would remain beyond the current shortage and would provide ongoing data about the nursing workforce as well as lead to strategies that would prevent future problems or quickly solve them.

The nursing and health care community has needed a comprehensive book on the nursing workforce. Cleary and Rice have summarized the work of Colleagues in Caring. With the other authors they provide the framework and the details that cities, regions, and states can use to provide the health care community with the data they need to decrease the cycles of shortages and surpluses that have plagued this country for years. Of course North Carolina is a model program and has had enormous success under Dr. Cleary's leadership. As a New Yorker I live in a state that does not have a state agency that deals with nursing workforce issues, nor is there one group that gathers the disparate data and forms a coherent picture of the nursing workforce. I hope RNs in New York can use the content of this book to work in that direction.

In times of shortages, the challenge is to separate those organizations that have a shortage because of poor management and/or working conditions including location and those organizations that have a shortage because there is a local, regional or national shortage. The Health Services and Resources Agency (HRSA) is working on meeting the challenge to identify shortage organizations that will benefit from HRSA's activities to relieve the RN shortage. HRSA must identify those organizations in which RNs who have benefited from Federal Funding of their educational expenses can fulfill their service obligation and/or have their loans forgiven. HRSA has asked the Center for Health Workforce Studies at the State University at Albany under the leadership of Jean Moore to identify criteria to identify these organizations. Content from this book will be enormously helpful as HRSA's effort goes forward over the next year.

While I expect that we will continue to have shortages and surpluses (although there are some people who only see shortages on the horizon) the content of this book, if read and used, will do much to decrease the intensity of these cyclical problems.

Preface

Past nursing workforce shortages have taught us that quick fixes are inadequate for addressing complex shortages. Without significant intervention involving long-range solutions, the current shortage promises to worsen dramatically over the next 20 years. The Robert Wood Johnson Colleagues in Caring Project led to a significant increase in nurse workforce planning and development at regional and state levels. Sustaining infrastructures for state level nursing workforce initiatives fosters greater understanding of nursing workforce issues and data-driven, comprehensive strategies and policy changes for nursing workforce development. *Nursing Workforce Development: Strategic State Initiatives* is designed to provide stakeholders with the latest information about nursing workforce centers, workforce data, and new education, workplace, and policy initiatives. The intended audience includes nursing leaders in education, service, health services research, and health policy. Also targeted are other stakeholders in the healthcare industry, workforce centers, and policy makers.

Chapter 1 provides a history of state nursing workforce initiatives in the United States, initiatives that demonstrated increasing organization and sophistication in the 1990s. Chapter 2 focuses on workforce development through leadership. Chapter 3 explores funding mechanisms and Chapter 4 focuses on workforce data. Chapters 5 and 6 describe the redesign of nursing work and simultaneous innovations in nursing education. Chapter 7 is policy focused and Chapter 8 portrays recruitment and retention efforts. Chapter 9 gives examples of state infrastructures for nursing workforce development that are demonstrating exponential growth in the current decade. The final chapter, Chapter 10, looks ahead into the future and next steps in this important work.

Acknowledgments

We acknowledge the work of a growing number of colleagues across the country who are committed to strategic nurse workforce planning. And we dedicate this book to Judy Seamon and Terry Keenan, visionaries and architects of the NC Center for Nursing and The Robert Wood Johnson Foundation Colleagues in Caring Program, respectively.

1

The Evolution of State Nursing Workforce Initiatives in the United States

Brenda Cleary and Rebecca Rice

INTRODUCTION: THE CONTEXT

Health care in the United States is in crisis. Unless changes are made, Medicare will go bankrupt within the next two decades as the U.S. population ages. Huge federal tax cuts, combined with a burgeoning federal deficit, indicate that there may be a general unwillingness in Congress to increase funding for most social programs and a desire to decrease commitments to entitlement programs. Even with steady federal and state funding, close to 41 million Americans are without health insurance at any one time. Furthermore, Healthy People 2010 indicators aim for elimination of health disparities for racial and ethnic peoples, but lack of funding may seriously interfere with achieving this worthy goal.

While the delivery system is in economic crisis, the health care workforce is heading toward a crisis of its own, and the most serious evidence of this is the nursing workforce. Nurses form the backbone of the health care delivery system. They are the largest number of health care providers (2.6 million). The nursing workforce is aging faster than the general population, and once the baby boomers, the largest cohort of nurses, begin to retire in 2008, the national demand for nurses will exceed the supply. Projections indicate that by 2020 there will be a national gap between supply and demand of minus 29 percent (U.S. Department of Health and Human Services, Health Resources and Services Administration, 2002).

Without sufficient numbers of experienced nurses, the quality and safety of the health care system are in jeopardy. Recent studies have demonstrated the linkages between mortality and morbidity rates and nurse staffing and the incidence of postoperative infections and numbers of registered nurses. Researchers have found significant relationships between nurse staffing levels and rates of urinary tract infections, pneumonia, upper gastrointestinal bleeding, and shock among hospitalized Medicare patients (Needleman, Buerhaus, Mattke, Stewart, & Zelevinsky, 2002). Their work confirmed earlier research showing that fewer nurses taking care of more patients is associated with a phenomenon called "failure to rescue," in which nurses who have too many patients are unable to conduct the surveillance necessary to prevent complications among hospitalized patients (Aiken, Clarke, Sloane, Sochalski, & Silber, 2002).

COLLEAGUES IN CARING: REGIONAL COLLABORATIVES FOR NURSING WORKFORCE DEVELOPMENT

Given the relationship between adequate numbers of nurses and the declining supply, stakeholders in nursing care have come together at regional, state, and national levels to engage in work aimed at resolving nursing workforce issues. Colleagues in Caring: Regional Collaboratives for Nursing Workforce Development, a program funded by The Robert Wood Johnson Foundation, catalyzed the formation of regional and statewide coalitions to examine nursing workforce issues.

Begun in 1996, the focus of Colleagues in Caring (CIC) was on regional and state levels, based on the premise that nursing workforce issues of supply and demand revolve around geographic labor markets. That is, nurses tend to be educated and to work in the same geographic area, and thus factors around the supply and demand for nurses are locally based. Hence, state nursing workforce coalitions serve as catalysts for local initiatives, advocating for state-based workforce supply and demand solutions and creating vehicles for the exchange of workforce information among regional labor markets (Prescott, 2000).

State-based nursing workforce entities are relatively new. In 1991, North Carolina became the first state to address a nursing shortage by passing legislation to create a state-funded Center for

Nursing. The ongoing activities of the North Carolina center focus on providing reports on the nursing workforce, convening groups to make recommendations about the nursing workforce, and developing and implementing an ongoing recruitment and retention program. The center has served as a model for the creation of other state-based initiatives. The North Carolina Center for Nursing is described in detail later in this chapter.

The CIC coalitions evaluated the capacity of the nursing workforce to meet the health care needs of the citizens, fostered programs that encouraged educational mobility among all levels of nursing education, promoted workplace initiatives for career advancement and satisfaction, and advocated for policies promoting nursing. The Robert Wood Johnson Foundation provided funding for 23 sites, and an additional 27 nonfunded states joined in nursing workforce development work. All 50 states and the District of Columbia have benefited from the wealth of nurse workforce expertise and innovative model development shared by network members.

CIC came along at the right time. In 1996 there was little discussion of a nursing shortage; in fact, the Pew Health Professions Commission (1995) had indicated that perhaps between 200,000 and 300,000 nursing positions would be lost as a result of a projected reduction in hospital beds. To wit, the commission had recommended closing and reducing nursing education programs by 10–20 percent. Simultaneously, the health care industry, primarily acute care hospitals, underwent extensive downsizing, rightsizing, and reengineering schemes, primarily to reduce labor costs. As a result of the tumultuous changes in work design, many experienced nurses left acute care for other less chaotic, more professionally rewarding health care settings. These nurses were replaced by less experienced nurses or unlicensed assistive personnel with little or no formal education. In this cycle of downsizing, reengineering, and replacement, CIC was born.

In the early CIC years, the main foci of the statewide coalitions were on collecting and analyzing nursing workforce data and evaluating competencies needed by the nursing workforce for making the transition into current and emerging practice sites. In the late 1990s, Buerhaus and his colleagues (Buerhaus, 1999; Buerhaus, Staiger, & Auerbach, 2000) were researching demographic trends in the nursing workforce, and instead of the predicted decline, they found an upward trend for demand and a slowly flattening supply curve well into the 21st century.

At the same time, CIC coalitions began to report shortages in some specialty areas such as critical care, emergency departments, and labor and delivery settings. Rather than continuing to focus on redeployment of nurses, they shifted their attention to developing and sharing recruitment strategies. The CIC National Program Office emerged as a hub for information on what the CIC sites were doing to meet nursing workforce needs. In addition, nonfunded states began to track into the CIC network, primarily through word-of-mouth. By its completion in 2003, CIC had grown to include almost all 50 states in its network.

Broadly viewed, the seven-year CIC program produced the following intended deliverables to the Robert Wood Johnson Foundation:

- Created and empowered regional and state collaboratives of nurse educators, employers of nurses, and other nursing stakeholders to take local responsibility for the widening gap between supply and demand for nurses and to take specific measurable actions to address the long-term, intransigent structural issues at the root of the U.S. shortage of nurses.

- Designed systems to collect regional- and state-based data on the supply, demand, and need dimensions of the nursing shortage; collaboratively conducting analyses of the data collaboratively by both employers and educators of nurses; and distributing and promoting the policy implications of the analyses to a wide variety of health care, academic, corporate, and governmental and health industry users.

- Helped to move the U.S. nursing education infrastructure to flexibility and utility by directly articulating all levels of nursing education from licensed practical nurse to graduate education. CIC's work enabled regions and states to move to a historically unprecedented national status by 2003, in which 31 regions or states now have educational mobility agreements involving over 500 nursing schools so that students with a wide variety of backgrounds and experiences can easily enter the nursing profession and rapidly and efficiently continue upward through the preparation levels of licensed and academic nursing programs.

- Directly influenced regional and state public policy debates and decisions regarding nursing workforce issues through a variety of skillful diplomatic and educational initiatives resulting in the creation in 2003 of 14 state centers for nursing workforce reports, legislation, forums, etc. That figure has now grown to 22 in 2004.

- Organized and conducted annual national meetings, attended by nursing leaders from almost all the states, that provided in-depth, rapid exchange of local and state information on nursing workforce issues and activities, unlike any other health industry national meetings.

Because of the deepening nursing shortage over the seven years of CIC's history, a clearer and more disturbing understanding of the implications of this shortage, and the explosive increase in the use of the Internet, the following unintended but equally impressive and compelling outcomes occurred:

- A new, locally based, but nationally linked and operative Internet-based "rapid response" system was created through CIC among nursing leadership in nursing associations, all levels of nursing education, and the entire continuum of employers of nurses.
- The identification, promotion, and mentorship of a new cadre of young nurse leaders accustomed and skilled in collaborative problem solving and decision making on behalf of the nursing profession with a CIC Internet-enabled capability to instantly communicate with each other, seek information and guidance, and access political networks of "friends of nursing" previously unavailable to them.
- The creation of new partnerships among regional and state nursing entities and other nursing stakeholders to engage their support and assistance in solving nursing shortage problems.
- Virtual teams of CIC nursing workforce innovators, locally based but nationally linked, able to provide consultations, presentations, and technical assistance in the following areas: nursing workforce research, recruitment and retention of nurses in a variety of workplace settings, nursing workforce data collection tools, analytic tools, report formatting, educational mobility agreements among all levels of schools of nursing, development of state nursing workforce centers, and economic modeling of nursing workforce issues.
- Evolution of an unprecedented national group of local/state funders with substantial combined levels of financial investment, committed to partnering with CIC in support of the future of the nursing profession.
- Use of the CIC collaboratives as contracting entities to perform studies for governments and academic institutions and to host forums.

- Creative, innovative brokering activities by the national program CIC staff among CIC projects and other local or national organizations committed to quality nursing care in the United States
- The presence of CIC nurse leaders in places, organizations, and roles as never before (national commissions, nongovernmental organizations' boards of directors, research enterprises, health care industry boards of trustees, and governmental agencies).

By 2003, 49 states were part of the CIC network. Table 1.1 lists the states involved in nursing workforce development work and identifies those that have been funded through the Robert Wood Johnson Foundation.

Unfortunately, the gap between supply and demand for nurses and nursing care has not diminished, although the state and regional nursing workforce coalitions have developed an array of effective initiatives aimed at narrowing that gap. FitchRatings (2003) foresaw "no relief to the current nursing shortage given increasing demand, an aging work force, and inadequate supply" (p. 7). Further, the financial institution states that this shortage will have a negative impact on the financial stability of health care institutions because these agencies will continue to search for and hire increasingly expensive health care workers with little guarantee that quality health care can be sustained in the unstable labor market (FitchRatings, 2003). Nursing leaders have the potential to contribute toward reversing the shortage, given continued coordination among diverse groups of nursing stakeholders.

THE FIRST PERMANENT INFRASTRUCTURE FOR NURSING WORKFORCE INITIATIVES

Enacting Policy: A Vision Becomes a Reality

Just as North Carolina was the first state to pass a nursing licensure law in 1903, in 1991, North Carolina became the first state to fund an agency dedicated to ensuring that there would be adequate nursing resources to meet the health care needs of its citizens. The vision was realized for the people of North Carolina when the 16 appointed members of the Board of Directors of the newly created Center for Nursing met for the first time on October 29, 1991. The creation of the North Carolina Center for Nursing was the culmination

Text continued on p. 10.

TABLE 1.1   States/Regions Participating in the Colleagues in Caring Network (2003)

State	Region or state	CIC funding (Y/N)	Comments
Alabama	State	N	
Alaska	State	Y	
Arizona	State	Y	
Arkansas	State	N	
California	State	Y	
Colorado	State	Y	
Connecticut	State	Y	
Delaware	State	N	
District of Columbia	Region	Y	
Florida	State	N	
Georgia	State	N	
Hawaii	State	Y	
Idaho	State	Y	
Illinois	State	N	
Indiana	Region/State	N	Two regional efforts are already in place, and a statewide initiative is forming.
Iowa	State	N	
Kansas	State	N	
Louisiana	Region/State	N	One regional effort underway in addition to a statewide effort.

(continued)

TABLE 1.1　States/Regions Participating in the Colleagues in Caring Network (2003) *(Continued)*

State	Region or state	CIC funding (Y/N)	Comments
Maine	State	N	
Maryland	State	Y	
Massachusetts	State	N	
Michigan	State	N	
Minnesota	State	Y	
Mississippi	State	Y	
Missouri	Region	Y (2)	Kansas City and Northeast regions.
Montana	State	Y	
Nebraska	State	N	
Nevada	State	N	
New Hampshire	State	N	
New Jersey	State	Y	
New Mexico	State	Y	
New York	Region	N	Regional educational initiatives underway.
North Carolina	State	Y	
North Dakota	State	N	

State	Region/State		Comments
Ohio	Region/State	Y	Four regional educational mobility regions; two workforce development regions.
Oklahoma	State	N	
Oregon	State	N	
Pennsylvania	Regions	N	Pittsburgh metro region.
Rhode Island	State	N	
South Carolina	Region/State	Y	Four geographic regions doing workforce initiatives with coordinated statewide effort.
South Dakota	State	Y	
Tennessee	State	Y	
Texas	Region	Y	Coastal Bend.
Utah	State	N	
Vermont	State	N	
Virginia	State	N	
Washington	State	N	
West Virginia	Region/State	Y	North Central region and statewide workforce development initiative underway.
Wisconsin	State	N	
Wyoming	State	N	

of three years of work by the North Carolina General Assembly and the Legislative Study Commission on Nursing. The Nursing Shortage Act of 1991 (GS 90-171) was the vehicle used to outline the mission and strategies defined by the legislature to address the nursing shortage that had plagued North Carolina in the late 1980s.

The North Carolina General Assembly created the Center for Nursing "to address issues of supply and demand for nursing, including issues of recruitment, retention, and utilization of nurse resources." The mission of the Center for Nursing is to ensure that the state has the nursing resources necessary to meet the health care needs of its citizens. Legislatively mandated goals include the following:

1. To develop a strategic statewide nursing workforce plan for North Carolina, addressing issues of supply and demand.
2. To convene various groups that include representatives from nursing, other health care professions, the business community, consumers, legislators, and educators to review the policy implications of the center's work.
3. To enhance and promote recognition, reward, and renewal activities for nurses in North Carolina through a comprehensive statewide recruitment and retention program.

The full impact of this legislative action is better understood in light of the budgetary challenges faced by the North Carolina legislature in 1991. In the 1989 to 1991 biennium, approximately $6.8 million was appropriated for nursing initiatives, including the establishment of the nursing scholars program. The North Carolina Nurse Scholars Program, modeled after the North Carolina Teaching Fellows Program, provided scholarships to attract the best and the brightest students into the nursing profession. When the $1.2 billion budget deficit became public knowledge, little hope was held for the implementation of the recommendations of the Legislative Study Commission on Nursing. Because of the deficit situation, the final report of the Legislative Study Commission on Nursing was submitted ahead of schedule in order to provide the general assembly with "timely information and recommendations." In the prelude to the final report, the cochairs of the Commission stated, "we believe that the recommendations are vital to continued programs in providing adequate health care for the future." When the general assembly adjourned, a $5.2 million appropriations bill had been passed including initial funding for the Center for Nursing of $341,200 for 1991–1992 and $460,000 for 1992–1993. The fact that a new initiative was funded, given the budgetary constraints, further affirmed the commitment of the general assembly to the health of the people of North Carolina and to the nurses who care for North Carolinians.

The Center for Nursing: The Early Years

During the inaugural meeting of the board of directors, the newly appointed board was greeted by the legislative counsel to the president pro tempore of the North Carolina Senate. Interestingly, in 1997, former President Pro Tempore Barnes was appointed to a three-year term on the board of directors for the center, bringing with him a unique and valued perspective on the history of the legislation that created the center. Also present during the first meeting were the senior fiscal analyst for the legislature and the vice president for finance for the University of North Carolina (UNC) general administration. The center maintains autonomy as a state agency; however, the center's budget resides under the UNC umbrella. This arrangement has been beneficial to the center because it removes budgetary and audit functions and provides human resources support for a very small state agency.

With the enabling legislation in place, the center was still a concept without real infrastructure. Judy Seamon, a politically astute nursing leader and a visionary who chaired the Legislative Study Commission Task Force for the Center of Excellence, was elected to serve as the first chair of the board of directors. The newly appointed board immediately began the work of establishing a new entity. From purchasing furniture to obtaining office space and hiring staff, board members volunteered to perform all the necessary activities under Mrs. Seamon's leadership. One of the first and most important functions of the board was the search for the executive director. Shirley Girouard, PhD, RN, FAAN, held the inaugural position and one by one, other staff positions were filled. Table 1.2 summarizes major accomplishments in the first five years of the center's existence.

Further Initiatives

Two of the legislative goals for the Center for Nursing, developing a statewide strategic plan and convening various stakeholders, were addressed by the North Carolina Nurse Workforce Planning Model. Implementation of the model was supported through a startup grant from The Duke Endowment, the center's state allocation,

TABLE 1.2   North Carolina Center for Nursing: The Early Years

1991   Center created by North Carolina General Assembly

1992   Initial board appointments; Judy Seamon, Chairperson
        Executive Director, Dr. Shirley Girouard, hired
        Center for Nursing locates at 3203 Woman's Club Drive in Raleigh
        Advisory Council formed
        Major data collection efforts underway

1993   First Trend Report on Nurse Supply released
        Institute for Nursing Excellence (INE) with Wake Area Health
            Education Center
        Directory of INE participants published
        Statewide survey of nurses in advanced practice and with
            advanced degrees
        Report to General Assembly
        Board appointments/reappointments (ongoing)

1994   School-based health care study released
        Evaluation of Nurse Scholars program released
        Represented on Data Collection/Info. Systems Committee of
            North Carolina Health Planning Commission
        Task Force on Workplace Issues initial report released
        Recognition, Reward & Renewal seed grant program (including
            dissemination workshop) established
        Executive Director, Dr. Brenda Cleary, hired
        Comprehensive report to General Assembly
        Profile of 1994 New Nursing Professionals released
        Report on Nurses with Advanced Degrees released

1995   Profile of Nurse Practitioners (NP) report released
        Trend Report on Nursing Supply 1982–93 released
        Follow-up report of Task Force on Workplace Issues
        Evaluation of Recognition, Reward and Renewal Grant Program
        Collaborative nurse workforce planning conference for Triangle
            and Mountain regions
        Subcontract with Research Triangle Institute on Health Care
            Financing Administration grant (NP care to Medicare
            recipients)
        Institute for Nursing Excellence in two sites, with support from
            Glaxo Wellcome
        Directory of all past INE participants produced
        First statewide nurse photo contest, sponsored by F&S Nursing
            Review Company and MedVisit, Inc.

(continued)

TABLE 1.2   *(Continued)*

Profile of 1995 new nursing professionals released
INE reunion seminar (Glaxo Wellcome sponsorship)
Volume 1, Issue 1 of NCCN newsletter disseminated
Expanded Advisory Council

1996   Center relocates to 222 N. Person Street in Raleigh
Fifteen new Recognition, Reward and Renewal grant projects
    implemented
Follow-up survey of 1995 nursing graduates completed
Health Care Recruiters Survey published
Distribution of nurse recruitment materials to public schools
    and media
Statewide nurse employer survey re: nursing demand
Dissemination of demand data in 9 AHEC regions
Introduction of North Carolina Nurse Workforce Planning Model;
    grant proposals developed
INE reunion seminar, combined with grant project dissemination,
    funded by Glaxo Wellcome
Survey of Advanced Practice Nurses to assess impact of 1993
    reimbursement legislation conducted

---

contributions from North Carolina hospitals and health systems, and phase II funding through the Robert Wood Johnson Foundation Colleagues in Caring Project.

Health policy bodies, such as the Pew Health Professions Commission, called for escalating health care workforce planning efforts. Nursing workforce issues are particularly complex, due to several factors. Nursing care, in both hospital and community-based settings, is provided by a range of personnel with varying levels of preparation from unlicensed assistive personnel to licensed practical nurses to registered nurses educated at the associate, baccalaureate, or graduate levels. Health care needs have never been greater. Growing numbers of elderly as well as other high-risk populations are often underinsured or uninsured. While hospital lengths of stay are shorter, acuity levels are higher. The Congressional Balanced Budget Act came on the heels of the health care industry's attempts to stabilize in light of the cost constraints of managed care. To ensure quality health services and desired outcomes in a health care system increasingly driven by marketplace economics and cuts in Medicare and Medicaid reimbursement, a ready and capable nursing workforce is critical.

The North Carolina Nurse Workforce Planning Model was conceived to assist hospitals and other health care agencies to meet evolving nursing resource demands. Development of the model involved initial conferences in each of the state's nine Area Health Education Center (AHEC) regions to disseminate state and intrastate regional information regarding supply and demand for nurses in North Carolina. Center for Nursing staff highlighted findings from the 1996 Survey of Nurse Employers (Cleary, Lacey, & Beck-Warden, 1998) with data analysis on a statewide and regional basis. The report described healthcare organizational changes in North Carolina affecting the demand among nurse employers for nursing personnel with differing levels of education and specific skills and competencies. The conferences provided not only a forum to disseminate data but an opportunity for regional experts to respond and comment as well, thus offering an additional qualitative perspective of regional applicability. Another purpose of these regional conferences was to provide startup guidance for regional nurse workforce planning groups in strategic planning initiatives.

Further evolution of regional alliances brought together nursing leaders from all levels of education and areas of practice to address local nursing issues in each of the state's nine AHEC regions. Annually, a statewide consortium component of the North Carolina Nurse Workforce Planning Model convened leaders from each regional planning alliance with nursing leaders at the state level, including the North Carolina Center for Nursing (the lead agency), the North Carolina Board of Nursing, the North Carolina Nurses Association, the North Carolina Licensed Practical Nurses Association, and the statewide AHEC nursing liaison as core members. Additional members included representatives from

- the North Carolina Department of Health and Human Services, Public Health Nursing
- the North Carolina Council of Deans and Directors of Baccalaureate and Higher Degree Programs
- the North Carolina Associate Degree Nursing directors
- North Carolina Practice Nurse educators
- the North Carolina Alliance of Hospital-Based Nursing Programs
- the North Carolina Organization of Nurse Executives
- the North Carolina Hospital Association
- the North Carolina Association for Home Care
- the North Carolina Health Care Facilities Association
- the North Carolina community college system

TABLE 1.3   North Carolina Statewide Plan for Nursing 2000

Goal 1: Create a dynamic statewide system for projecting nurse workforce demand.

Appraise population demographic and health indicator data available in North Carolina as they influence demand for nursing services.

Project how changes in the health care delivery system, including the use of technology, will affect nursing demand in terms of numbers and educational mix.

Evaluate the North Carolina Nursing CareerLine as a viable tool for assessing current demand and for tracking developing trends.

Study relationships between various staffing models and patient outcomes.

Goal 2: Ensure an adequate nursing workforce for North Carolina, in terms of numbers, ethnic diversity, educational mix, and geographic distribution.

Monitor nurse workforce supply trends through secondary analysis of data from the North Carolina Board of Nursing and the Division of Facility Services.

Develop creative mechanisms to attract a diverse group of students to nursing as an attractive and viable career option.

Develop strategies for ensuring adequate numbers of faculty who are prepared to mentor students in a changing health care system.

Further develop articulation options at the baccalaureate and graduate level that recognize previous learning and experience and are distributed throughout the state. Monitor educational program data (e.g., applications, enrollments, and graduate outcomes).

Provide resources and programs (formal mechanisms) designed to promote recognition and retention.

Goal 3: Promote collaboration between nursing education and practice to determine necessary competencies and design professional practice.

Continue to support and develop collaboratives of nursing education and practice at the regional and state level.

Provide funding for the planning and implementation of demonstration projects of professional practice models, with an emphasis on differentiated practice.

- the North Carolina university system
- the North Carolina Association of Independent Colleges and Universities

Implementation of the North Carolina Nurse Workforce Planning Model resulted in the development of a statewide plan for nursing in North Carolina, which may be found in Table 1.3. Workforce planning cannot be considered an automatic fix for the prevention of nursing shortages because cycles of shortages are complex phenomena. However, a more strategic approach to ensuring adequate nursing personnel to meet health care industry demands and citizens' needs has resulted in North Carolina maintaining one of the lowest vacancy rates for RNs in the country. Systematic, long-range planning also enhances communication between nursing service providers and nursing educators in the qualitative aspect of planning and development, particularly regarding nursing competencies needed now and in the future.

The North Carolina Center for Nursing is a visible commitment to the criticality of nursing resources and fulfills its mission by (1) providing objective information to health care providers, policy makers, and other stakeholders; (2) developing a strategic planning mechanism for nursing resources in North Carolina; and (3) promoting recruitment and retention by recognizing and rewarding excellence and ensuring recognition among nurse colleagues. The Center for Nursing is an exciting innovation and can serve as a model for other states.

2

Leadership Development

Joyce Clifford, Michael Bleich,
Peggy O'Neill Hewlett, Edith Irving,
and Cynthia Armstrong Persily

"Leadership is much more an art, a belief, a condition of the heart, than a set of things to do. The visible signs of artful leadership are expressed ultimately, in its practice."
— Max De Pree, *Leadership is an Art,* 1985

A CALL TO DEVELOPING CURRENT AND FUTURE LEADERS IN NURSING

Even in a world of dramatic change and perceived chaos, there remain certain factors considered constants. For nursing, the concepts of caring, commitment, and collaboration come to mind immediately, and even the notion of change itself rates high on the list of things that nurses can count on and will be expected to manage and bring into the context of a caring relationship with patients, families, and communities. Another nursing constant is the search and frequently expressed need for leadership, which relates in large part to the nursing profession's ever-present goal: excellence in nursing practice.

The work of leaders is often hidden, only becoming clear when events are examined fully. Leaders emerge from a set of intertwined events and also work in a web of interconnecting events. Hegelsen (1995) aptly described the web of relationships that many consider an essential core element for successful leadership. This chapter provides examples of the importance of building relationships in order to achieve desired outcomes. Other writers focus on the leader as a visionary, suggesting that leaders see opportunities and are prepared to act even when they may not have planned to do so.

Benner and associates wrote that leaders have an intuitiveness that helps them make connections and take action (Benner, Tanner, & Chesla, 1996).

Leadership is often thought of as being positional, as part of an organization's hierarchy. That is, certain positions within an organization are considered to be the leader positions. These positional leaders are often thought to have both special rights and obligations as a result of this level of organizational recognition and accountability. Some positions embody an inherent level of organizational leadership that is obligatory. In nursing, however, leaders can be found everywhere—in the formal leadership roles such as those in management, administration, education, etc., as well as in the variety of clinical roles traditionally found in most health care organizations such as clinical staff nurses, nurse specialists, nurse educators, and many others. Recognizing and supporting these leadership roles enhance the opportunity to ensure positive outcomes and the ultimate goal of providing superb clinical care. In essence, all nurses who consider themselves professionals should also consider themselves leaders. To do any less is a disservice to the populations that nurses seek to serve and the health organizations in which they practice.

The capacity for leadership is an intrinsic component of professionalism, and the need to develop this capacity is an obligation of the individual as well as the profession. Leadership development should be highly valued and embraced by all. As professionals, nurses must accept the responsibility to assume leadership roles not only within an organization but through the spectrum of professional activities that call for leadership in shaping multiple health care and societal issues. Part of our social responsibility as professionals is to ensure that there are many points of influence, many leaders, who can engage in the myriad changes that are now confronting society, including changing economics, demographics, technology, and health policy. For leadership effectiveness to occur, those in the front lines of care delivery must be as well prepared and empowered as leaders as are those in the executive suites of hospitals, universities, and public offices.

Just as leadership can be defined from a broad perspective and from a more conventional perspective of positional leadership, so can the development of leaders be defined. Formal programs of leadership development provided by professional educators and continuing education services are often used to develop staff in leadership positions. But mentoring and sponsorship are also important aspects of developing individuals. The next generation of nurse leaders depends on the current generation to help shape the future for them, that is, to help new nurse leaders develop their ability to continue the legacies of past leaders and to develop skills that will help them create new leadership outcomes. It is incumbent on all nurse professionals to accept personal responsibility for helping to shape the leadership of the next generation. As stated by Peters, "Leadership is ultimately an act of faith in other people" (Peters, 2002).

Leadership development includes preparing the nurse professional to lead in complex environments, setting direction and helping others see the vision encapsulated in that direction, making collaborative decisions, and communicating them effectively across a myriad of relationships that the leader has developed, nurtured, and promoted. The attributes of effective leaders are well known: personal competence, effective communication, wisdom in risk-taking, creativity in thought and action, and—without exception—consistent integrity that generates trust and respect from others.

Role modeling and actions such as those exemplified by the Colleagues in Caring initiatives described in this chapter help establish a framework for operationalizing leadership actions and outcomes. The potential for real influence in the health care system has grown in direct proportion to the depth of knowledge and breadth of activities required of the nursing profession and its leaders. The Colleagues in Caring program provides multiple and exceptional examples of such leadership.

DEFINITIONS

"All men dream: but not equally. Those who dream by night in the dusty recesses of their minds wake in the day to find that it was vanity: but the dreamers of the day are dangerous men, for they may act their dream with open eyes to make it possible."
—T. E. Lawrence, *Seven Pillars of Wisdom*

Although leadership development was not a stated objective of the Robert Wood Johnson Foundation's Colleagues in Caring (CIC) program, the nature of CIC initiatives and the amalgamation of novice to experienced individuals working collaboratively made leadership development a positive and significant consequence of CIC. For many, the CIC structure and activities created local, regional, and national opportunities for individuals to create and share strategies to influence workforce development and improve work environments. The commingling of a strong mission based on shared values and concerns, a framework to work from but not rigidly prescribed, acknowledgment of regional variations that encouraged creative and innovative solutions, and blending intellectual and material capital from service, academia, and other sources was exactly the platform from which participants could exercise and evolve their leadership, management, and followership skills.

Leadership, as used here, reflects the use of personal traits and power to constructively and ethically influence others to an endpoint vision or goal. Exact or predictable steps to achieve the goal are not known, must be decided along the way, or require adaptation from what is known. The essence of leadership is relationship based and principle driven and requires the communication of direction and reasonable risk-taking with an air of self-assuredness that evokes confidence in others (Bleich, 2003). Leadership was essential to each CIC initiative. New territory was forged to create best practice models to (a) prepare a qualified workforce to meet the imminent and amplified challenges from increased consumer demand and expectations, and (b) to enhance antiquated care delivery models and improve challenging work environments.

The meaning of *management* differs, but it evolves from effective leadership. Leaders forge into the unknown to create change, and at some point this change becomes systematized, based on newly established norms, expectations, and outcomes (Bleich, 2003). In some ways, effective management is more challenging than effective leadership because the excitement often associated with leadership ventures requires tenacity and repetition in management. The model that guided the CIC initiatives fostered leadership through innovation and creativity but also recognized the need for management because sustainability of change was fostered and expected. Sustainability, then, requires management.

CIC amassed a vast number of new, talented, and committed individuals who had the common goal of improving the nursing workforce and the work environment. Effective leadership and management guided and, ultimately, standardized and sustained change. However, without followers, CIC project leaders would never have achieved the major objectives. *Followership* refers to the behaviors demonstrated by the individuals with whom the leader or manager interacts. Followership is the healthy, assertive use of personal behaviors that contribute directly to the vision and objectives and is sometimes confused as passivity or taking directions without thought. This is not the case. Followers *acquiesce* to leaders in certain tasks, such as direction setting, politicking, pacesetting, or planning (Bleich, 2003).

Images of leading, managing, and following often focus—inappropriately—on roles and hierarchical structures. In fact, every individual involved in CIC brought to the table his or her personal capacity for leading, managing, and following. During any interaction, individuals stepped up to the plate and fluidly moved between leadership, management, and followership roles, partly out of personal preference but also out of necessity. Structures that promulgated hierarchical behaviors were minimized, thereby enhancing individual opportunities to practice leading, managing, and following.

A brief discussion of the concept of collaboration is in order. Collaboration demands that individuals possess the skills and abilities in each domain and shift easily between them. Collaboration was a strong philosophical foundation for all CIC activities, but the concept that has lost definitional crispness with common use over time, contributing to misconceptions and differences among health care practitioners about the meaning of the term (Gardner, 1998). Derived from a concept analysis conducted by Kinnaman (1999), *collaboration* is defined by Kinnaman and Bleich (2004) as a "communication process among individuals who (a) are of differing disciplines or organizational rank, (b) band together for advanced problem solving, (c) discern innovative solutions without regard to discipline or rank, and (d) enact change based on a higher standard of care or organizational practice. The process requires mutual respect, differing but complementary competencies, a distributive balance of power between the parties, and evidence of satisfying teamwork resulting in change" (p. 311). Collaboration is often confused with cooperation or coordination, or even tolerance. Suffice it to say that complex problem solving is best served by collaboration. The nursing workforce and work environment are complex issues.

Based on this definition, CIC was a collaborative venture. The workforce and work environment examples in this book demonstrate the variety of stakeholders who came together, regardless of varying organizational roles and ranks. Local variation and need were recognized and celebrated, thereby promoting innovative solutions and advanced problem solving. Complementary competencies created new models for enacting change in curricula, recruitment strategies, care delivery, or work environment. Feedback loops, a key function of the program staff, were built into the process, and this ensured sharing of best practices between projects, which led to a higher standard of care. Respect for the similarities and differences between service and academia grew as all parties "heard the voice" of each stakeholder. In summary, the collaboration fostered throughout CIC initiatives enriched leaders' capacity to lead, managers' capacity to manage, and followers' effective function in full and active partnership.

CORE LEADERSHIP COMPETENCIES FOR TODAY AND THE FUTURE

Any successful initiative requires leaders who have learned from the past so they can better forecast the future. Transformations such as those necessary to ensure an adequate future nursing workforce will only occur if leaders are present at all levels—national, regional, state, professional, and institutional—to capitalize on opportunities to enhance the workforce and the workplace and to move the profession forward, making the most of those opportunities (O'Neil & Coffman, 1998). The work of conceptualizing, implementing, evaluating, and sustaining statewide nursing workforce centers has sought, and continues to seek leaders who have internalized five core leadership competencies: self-knowledge, strategic vision, risk-taking and creativity, interpersonal and communication, effectiveness, and inspiring and leading change—form the basis for leading in an environment in which massive transformation is occurring and will continue to be necessary (Robert Wood Johnson Executive Nurse Fellows Program, 2003).

Self-Knowledge

Self-knowledge connotes individuals' ability to understand themselves in the context of organizational challenges, interpersonal demands, and individual motivation (Robert Wood Johnson Executive Nurse Fellows Program, 2003). Knowledge of self involves careful and planned introspection and allows more fully realized personal values, strengths, and responsibilities. Self-knowledge enhances leaders' abilities to judge when to lead and when to follow, essential skills for participants in the statewide nursing workforce movement.

One author experienced this firsthand when leading the effort to advance legislation to create a nursing workforce center in her home state. While she was an expert in statewide nursing workforce issues, she competently reflected that she was not the expert to lead the legislative process. In essence, this left two choices—to forge ahead, learning the legislative process and risking failure in working the issue through the legislature, or to promote success by contracting with someone with complementary talents who was already an expert in the legislative process and known as a successful lobbyist/leader in representing nursing and women's issues in the legislature. The author's reflective understanding of her strengths and her recognition that a leader motivates and inspires others to add their expertise to the situation at hand exemplifies the importance of knowing when to lead and when to follow (or, as in this case, when to work collaboratively), and ultimately ensured success in the legislative process.

Strategic Vision

Strategic vision is the ability to connect broad social, economic, and political changes to the strategic direction of institutions and organizations (Robert Wood Johnson Executive Nurse Fellows Program, 2003). A strategic vision is a mental model for a desired future state. Like self-knowledge, this competency involves thinking about the future within the context of the present and past, and then developing and communicating the image of the aspired future.

The history of the statewide nursing workforce center movement exemplifies the importance of having a strategic vision and, in retrospect, shows how this vision was integral to the growth of the movement. Workforce leaders envisioned their future as reflected in the following scenario. In 1991, North Carolina became the first state to fund an agency dedicated to ensuring the adequacy of nursing resources to meet the health care needs of its citizens. When the 16-member Board of Directors for the North Carolina Center for Nursing met for their first meeting, the vision was realized, the culmination of a three-year effort by the North Carolina General Assembly and the Legislative Study Commission on Nursing. The Nursing Shortage Act of 1991 outlined the mission and strategies defined by the legislature to address nursing shortage issues that had plagued North Carolina since the late 1980s.

Now, the challenge is to manage and sustain the vision. The compelling vision is that "the North Carolina Center for Nursing will be a recognized leader in nurse workforce research, long-range planning and policy development, and comprehensive recruitment and retention efforts" and pursue innovation and excellence to "serve as a model for similar initiatives throughout the nation and the world" (North Carolina Center for Nursing, 2004). Enacting a vision such as this requires leadership, management, and followership.

Risk-Taking and Creativity

In their simplest form, risk-taking and creativity are the abilities to transform the self and the organization by moving outside of traditional and patterned ways of success (Robert Wood Johnson Executive Nurse Fellows Program, 2003). All leaders must take risks in order to lead: trying new behaviors, abandoning what they do well to explore what they know less well, and developing new models to achieve their missions. Examples of risk-taking and creativity in the statewide nursing workforce movement abound. Each statewide center broke through boundaries to promote communication, data exchange, and articulation arrangements among the various levels of nursing education, service and education settings, and service, education, and government organizations.

An example of is the collaborative work of the Arizona Hospital and Health Care Association. In 1996, the Arizona Hospital and Healthcare Association (AzHHA) received the Arizona CIC grant to establish the Healthcare Institute (HCI). The primary mission of the HCI was and is to provide workforce advocacy for members of AzHHA. The Arizona CIC grant was committed to "enhancing the health and welfare of Arizonans by improving access to a nursing work force prepared to meet evolving consumer healthcare needs and consumer demands" (Arizona Hospital and Healthcare Association, 2004).

To meet specific goals, such as developing a regional and statewide educational articulation program, arrangements were fostered among educational and service institutions to initiate leadership development and professional advocacy programs and establish data systems to capture and forecast workforce data. Leaders realized that functioning in isolation was stifling progress and that forging mutual trust relationships was essential to move forward creatively.

Interpersonal and Communication Effectiveness

Interpersonal and communication effectiveness requires skill in translating strategic vision into compelling and motivating messages (Robert Wood Johnson Executive Nurse Fellows Program, 2003). Visioning a desired future is not enough. A strategic vision is a focused and clear message, regardless of the complexity of the issue being addressed. A compelling, clearly understood vision can be enacted with enthusiasm and goal orientation. Building interpersonal relationships and providing feedback through the evaluation process helped each of the CIC projects develop their respective messages to serve as an impetus for change.

At West Virginia University, the CIC project led the effort to bring together leaders from health care facilities, service providers, and education in the north central region of West Virginia to analyze nurse retention in this rural state. An early initiative was the sensitive issue of surveying nurse employers and working nurses about factors that influenced retention and nurses' intent to stay in or leave a position and/or an organization.

The results revealed a serious mismatch between the long-held beliefs of health care executives (that nurses wanted improved salaries, benefits, and parking) and the actual wants and needs of working nurses for respect, autonomy, flexibility, and recognition. Since the view of health care executives drove the institutional initiatives for retention of nurses, successful and sensitive development of a communication plan and presentation of a cogent message about the study results were urgent.

The CIC participants shaped their message and showed sensitivity to the various cultures and stakeholders using a variety of communication methods to reach constituents throughout the state. The strategy to present the information in a "quietly persistent" manner was successful, and the message was launched repeatedly at numerous local professional meetings, institutional gatherings, chambers of commerce meetings, and individual meetings with human resource directors and health care executives. Complementing these face-to-face approaches—the critical link for West Virginians—were written and electronic reinforcements of the message, such as brochures, publications, and a Web-site. The final result of this quietly persistent communication plan was an increased awareness of the need for the kind of change in the work environment that was more congruent with the desires of staff nurses.

Inspiring and Leading Change

The final competency is inspiring and leading change. It is key to leadership effectiveness. The ability to create, structure, and effectively implement organizational change in a continuous manner is crucial not only in the creation of statewide nursing workforce centers but also in the ongoing management tasks required to sustain these centers. True leaders of change must be able to overcome resistance, broker power, and negotiate solutions. Mississippi's CIC project epitomized how a group of nursing leaders inspired and led change in their state.

The Mississippi CIC initiative emerged from a platform built by nursing organizations over a 13-year period, bringing together nursing leaders to address core issues related to public policy and the workforce/work environment. About 25 entities were represented in the Nursing Organization Liaison Committee (NOLC) conceived by the Mississippi Nurses Association (MNA). The NOLC is composed of all Mississippi nursing education programs; an eclectic group of nursing employers from hospital, home care, and community settings; regulators of nurses and health care organizations; professional associations; consumers of health services; and payers. Nurse leaders from these entities were power brokers noted for their collective success in influencing legislation on all issues related to the profession. When change was indicated, these leaders were called into action to orchestrate grassroots involvement. In essence, the NOLC exemplifies a political machine capable of coalescing individual efforts into a successful change team.

Through the efforts of the MNA and the NOLC, the state's legislature passed and partially funded the Nursing Workforce Redevelopment Act during the 1996 session, during a "no new appropriations" session. The Act authorized the Mississippi Board of Nursing to establish the Office of Nursing Workforce (ONW) that would be responsible for addressing changes affecting the nursing workforce.

This broad-based coalition of change agents, the NOLC, created the model for what became one of the most innovative and successful nursing workforce initiatives in the country. Mississippi's nursing leaders, understanding the impact of federal budget cuts and the developing managed care market, crafted a visionary plan to prepare and maintain a competent nursing workforce to ensure effective patient care delivery. The philosophy driving the ONW initiative was that the health and welfare of the people of Mississippi required a highly competent nursing workforce. To meet this challenge, accurate data on nursing supply and demand were required to inform change activities and influence health policy makers and planners. Wisely, this group understood that workforce planning and redevelopment required action based on reliable annual data obtained through the CIC project. The challenge for all statewide nursing workforce centers is to move leadership in theory to leadership in action.

BRINGING CORE LEADERSHIP COMPETENCIES TOGETHER

The preceding scenarios support the premise that CIC grant recipients were composed of committed individuals who shared leadership, management, and followership opportunities to improve the workforce and the workplace. Further, the application of core leadership competencies, specified above (self-knowledge, strategic vision, risk-taking and creativity, interpersonal and communication effectiveness, and inspiring and leading change) was manifested repeatedly as centers collaborated to benefit care for the citizens who count on nursing care to meet far-reaching health care needs. The description that follows is yet another example of leadership in action.

The Idaho Commission on Nursing and Nursing Education (ICNNE) learned firsthand the revolutionary value of leadership by transforming a loosely structured volunteer organization into a structured virtual network, using technology to span the vast distances of this rural state. The virtual organization became a productive network of individuals who developed ongoing electronic media to conduct business when traditional in-person communication was deemed impractical.

ICNNE began the journey in 1966 as a major force in framing issues for nurses in the state. This group served as the focal point for generating systemic responses to nursing education and workforce concerns. ICNNE provided the structure for leaders of Idaho's health care employers, nursing associations, and nine nursing schools to address nursing issues, thus building on its long history of encouraging collaboration among diverse stakeholders.

In 1995 the role of the ICNNE shifted when it was contacted by the Idaho State Board of Education and the State Board of Nursing about hotly contested political discussions about entry into practice. ICNNE was contracted to conduct a statewide study to determine the nursing competencies of each level of practice and the validity of defined education levels. In delineating competencies, ICNNE systematically assessed the state's current and projected nursing workforce needs across all health care settings. Once competencies and supply-and-demand projections were articulated, ICNNE was to determine whether the existing capacity and infrastructure were sufficient to meet the identified health care needs of the citizenry. ICNNE conducted these studies, which became known as the Idaho Nursing Workforce and Strategic Planning Project. Closely matching the goals and project activities completed by participants in the Robert Wood Johnson CIC projects (Phase One), this project differed in that it was, at this point, entirely funded from the private sector.

With assistance from a project consultant, ICNNE undertook a three-pronged research approach. First, it assessed what other states with a similar cultural milieu were doing in workforce development. Second, ICNNE determined employer attitudes toward the future nursing workforce. Third, ICNNE measured the attitudes of Idaho nurses about future workforce issues and whether their educational preparation adequately prepared them for practice.

With volunteer efforts from nurse leaders in practice and education throughout the state, new and creative methods of gathering research information were tested. Nurse stakeholders truly collaborated and led the effort when necessary, but they also acquiesced to become engaged followers who worked instead of just advising. Seeing its goal-directed results achieved, ICNNE members committed to work together in pursuit of other workforce solutions. In 1999, ICNNE was selected as a site for the second round of CIC funding.

In this second round of CIC funding, ICNNE leaders identified from their research findings a major competency gap for nurses: a lack of management/leadership preparation in both academic and service settings. Employers in small, rural settings lamented the lack of expertise and/or financial resources to provide leadership training. Responsively, ICNNE undertook the development of the Idaho Nursing Leadership Network, whose purpose was to provide education to all levels of nurse leaders throughout the state. The financial resources to support this project came from the CIC grant and a Murdock Charitable Trust Grant. The ICNNE Nursing Leadership Network was inaugurated in January 2001.

Once again, a virtual network was used as the vehicle to provide educational offerings and to parse out the work assignments required to create the educational product. The network's members met face-to-face twice, early on to develop consensus about the goals and objectives to be achieved and at completion to evaluate the results of having implemented the Nursing Leadership Network.

Through the network, management courses for beginning supervisors and mid-level managers were developed using a contracted "content author" who was guided by the strategic vision and directives established by an oversight steering committee. The steering committee members served as content editors and approved final content. The courses were piloted with over 100 participants in three diverse locations across Idaho in fall 2001, followed by course refinements.

The following year, a standardized curriculum for three levels of nurse leadership was piloted across the state and met with phenomenal success. Courses were offered from three primary sites, and distance-learning augmented on-site learning for rural communities. Participants opted to take these courses for academic credit or for continuing education units. If taken for academic credit, all nursing schools agreed to accept these credits in a portfolio program leading to an advanced degree. Gaining consensus for this program from each nursing school was no small task, but it was plausible to overcome institutional barriers to foster leadership advancement. The vision, with buy-in from stakeholders who took risks to model new collaborative behavior, sent a strong message to nurses that serious efforts to improve the work environment were real. The effort was reinforced locally and disseminated nationally when an article appeared in *Patient Care Management* entitled, "Providing Leadership in Rural Health Care: The Evolving Role of Virtual Teams in Managing Projects" (Robinson, 2003).

The journey did not end there. In fall 2003, ICNNE entered a formal partnership with the Idaho Organization of Nurse Executives (IONE). The organizations had common missions, visions, goals, and objectives regarding nursing-related workforce issues and the profession. Not surprisingly, the virtual network is being used in this new partnership to reach all of the members across the state. A joint governing board has been established and the work begun by the commission now includes the newly created Idaho Nursing Workforce Center. Areas of focus are leadership, workforce issues, and education, including fine-tuning the state's articulation agreement. Efforts are underway to create a foundation to provide grant funding to hospitals to enhance bedside nursing. Initial funding is from money donated by each organization and supplemented by state funding.

What started as a diverse group of leaders rallying around a core need has evolved into a strong and structured collaborative process that will outlast the success of one project. Nursing leaders have modeled the attributes they are seeking to develop in new nurses and infuse into the profession as a whole.

The lessons learned during the Idaho journey were not easy, but each accomplishment brought energy and evidence that leaders make a difference. Leaders learned to step outside their individual comfort zones and envision what was best for the citizens and the profession, not just their own arena of practice or educational role. Personal agendas and politics were set aside after months of painful "storming." The greater good became the driving force that transformed volunteer leaders from a group of individuals representing diverse agendas and settings into an impressive leadership alliance.

It cannot be overlooked that regardless of desire and dedication to a common goal, nursing leaders in Idaho were volunteers already beset with organizational responsibilities. To turn dreams into action required a paid, dedicated director/coordinator to organize, implement, and manage, the work that turned dreams into reality.

The commission and IONE consist of strong individual leaders who have become a team in which control is shared. Leaders must be strong and willing to step forward when needed, and then step back to be a follower and let others take the lead. This ability to oscillate was one of the most difficult lessons learned. The passion for the vision must not overshadow the expediency of getting things done, even if results lack perfection. Continuous improvement will be the work ahead for future leaders.

NEXT STEPS IN THE LEADERSHIP JOURNEY

In summary, the leadership lessons of the statewide nursing workforce movement are many and form the basis of future challenges. The initiatives described above demonstrate the importance of fluid movement through leadership, management, and followership roles. One cannot overstate the importance of stretching beyond comfort levels, of stepping outside of what is "good for me" to look at what is good for the group, of developing a strategic vision of what could be or taking a risk to create change, and of careful planning, analysis, and evaluation. Collaboration, team development, and leveraging relationships are continued challenges for leaders in the nursing workforce development movement.

Leading Into the Future

The Robert Wood Johnson Foundation CIC initiative will stand as a significant nursing workforce program in the history of the profession. The key to success in this project seems to be how the core objectives resonated with staff nurses, nurse educators, and employers. Nurses and others now realize more than ever before that essential nursing care is what individuals seek when they go to hospitals and other clinical settings and that, without nurses, the health of the public is at risk. The CIC leaders envisioned this far ahead of the current shortage and wisely stimulated state and regional collaborative partnerships to jump-start the generation of solutions to stave off the impending crisis.

The objectives of the national program empowered and enabled nurse leaders across all sectors of the profession to join hands and address the multiple dimensions of issues influencing the nursing shortage. This approach stimulated bridging and overcoming the historical splits among the country's nurses. Stakeholders were identified from nursing and beyond, creating a leadership base with a broad focus.

Twenty states were awarded initial Robert Wood Johnson Foundation funding, and three additional states joined Phase II of the program. Before the projects officially ended, more than 35 states had CIC-like initiatives up and running. The success of the program can be strongly linked to leaders found at local, state, and regional levels. Grassroots groups were funded and empowered to create systems that addressed the needs of local constituencies but centered on the national core objectives. This created synergy to do the right work for the right reasons. The national program office coordinated the efforts and created links to the local and state groups, allowing solutions to emerge and be shared when relevant. At annual sponsored meetings by the Robert Wood Johnson Foundation, the different strategies to address workforce and work environment issues were shared, and nurses from various regions of the country learned about issues, shared what was working in their areas, found collegial support to keep the momentum alive, and created webs of influence.

O'Neil (2004) stated that developing successful teams is a critical element of leadership. He outlines three types of teams: oversight teams, operational teams, and task teams. In retrospect, it is evident that these team types were present in the most successful CIC projects. Nursing leaders' ability to identify talented people to include in the teams and along with their clear understanding and utilization of leadership, management, and followership strategies were keys to success.

The CIC projects were not designed to focus on leadership development, but the need to develop leaders became strikingly evident as funding ended and the need for sustainability became imperative. The CIC projects created a cadre of nursing leaders, never before seen, in the areas of workforce and work environment. Many of these nurses are now nationally noted experts in various sectors of workforce issues.

To position the nursing discipline at the national level, new leaders need to be mentored and groomed to lead the state nursing workforce initiatives still underway. Bleich, Hewlett, Santos, Rice, Cox, and Richmeier (2003) called upon all nursing leaders to do the following:

- Address the problems and solutions requiring nationally orchestrated strategies.
- Recognize that shortages require localized strategies.
- Recognize that each nurse is called to involvement.

As Gary Hamel stated, "the goal is not to speculate on what might happen; but to imagine what you can make happen" (Robert Wood Johnson Foundation Executive Nurse Leader Fellows meeting, October 2001, Chicago). Simply put, there is an impending public health crisis because there are not enough nurses. Experienced nurses are leaving the field, and fewer people want to go into it. The result is that the public's health is at risk. And nursing leaders from the Colleagues in Caring program and all the state nursing workforce centers have a primary role to play in addressing these critical issues.

3

Funding Nursing Workforce Coalitions or How to Find Your Sugar Daddy

Judith Kline Leavitt

T he most creative and innovative goals for any workforce coalition cannot be accomplished without money. Coalitions need funding not only for planning but also for sustainability. Since funding is so critical, this chapter focuses on ways to secure funding. Information about securing public funds, particularly through legislative and regulatory grants, is compared with funding from the private sector. Two sources—state workforce funds and hospital conversion foundations—are discussed more extensively because of their potential as funding streams that are new and relatively untapped by nursing workforce coalitions. To ensure sustainability, nursing workforce coalition leaders must secure funding from a variety of sources. The more creative coalitions are in securing funds from different sources, the better workforce initiatives will be at withstanding changes in economic conditions. The goal for any workforce coalition is to find a Sugar Daddy!

LEGISLATIVE INITIATIVES

State workforce coalitions' most commonly sought funding mechanism when establishing nursing centers and workforce projects has been state legislatures appropriations. North Carolina was the first state (1991) to establish a legislatively mandated entity to study workforce trends and initiate recruitment and retention strategies. In March 2003, Mary Lou Brunell, Director of the Florida Center for Nursing, and Rebecca Rice, Deputy Director of Colleagues in

Caring, conducted a telephone survey of the 13 centers then in existence to ascertain how they were funded. Just like North Carolina, most were funded through state legislatures, at least initially (Brunell & Rice, 2003). As the nursing shortage worsened in 2004, more state legislatures provided funding to get centers started, and by 2004, 19 states had appropriated state funding for state workforce projects.

Depending on the administrative structure of the workforce entity, funding can go directly to the center (as in North Carolina) through an annual appropriation by the legislature or to an administrative unit that has jurisdiction over the office. For instance, in Mississippi, the funding goes through the board of nursing, under which the Mississippi Office of Nursing Workforce (MONW), is placed. The funding is allocated annually and is designated for the MONW and cannot be used by the board for other needs. In other states, such as Florida and New Mexico, funding may only be designated to initiate a project, with no assurance of long-term support. A few states, such as Alaska, South Dakota, and Tennessee, have passed legislation that funds workforce centers through licensing fees or car tags. Such innovative mechanisms can ensure long-term funding.

Legislative appropriations reflect coalitions' effectiveness in making their needs known to policy makers. In a time of shrinking state resources, such funding becomes difficult to obtain. Appropriations are usually made on an annual basis. As a result, consistent lobbying by workforce supporters is necessary to garner funding. Unless funding is tied into a multiyear authorization, annual legislative appropriations tend to be less secure than other funding sources.

PUBLIC GRANTS

U.S. Department of Health and Human Services

Public funding at the federal level comes primarily through the Health Resources and Service Administration (HRSA) in the Department of Health and Human Services. Many of the grants are used to expand educational opportunities for students in baccalaureate and graduate programs through traineeships and fellowships. Congressional directives mandate particular emphasis on recruitment of minorities and under-represented groups into the health professions. Because of the shortage of some health professionals, especially nurses, new funding streams focus on innovative projects for recruitment and retention. For example, in May 2004, a proposal was initiated for Health Careers Adopt a School Demonstration Programs (HCSDP). The purpose of the HCSDP program was to stimulate the development of partnerships between community-based organizations, schools, and health professionals to increase the interest, preparation, and pursuit of health careers among under-represented minority (URM) and disadvantaged students. HRSA sought models that can be replicated and utilized by schools (middle and high school), community-based organizations, and other educational or health-related entities.

Much information about grant proposals can be found at the HRSA Website (http://www.hrsa.gov/grants/preview/default.htm). Proposal announcements change frequently, and there is often a short time frame for completing applications so check the Website on a regular basis.

U.S. Department of Labor

The U.S. Department of Labor is a significant resource for information about the workforce such as employment statistics, labor rules and regulations, and workforce grants. The newest area for workforce grant funding is known as the Employment and Training Administration. This initiative, introduced by President George W. Bush in 2003, aims to provide direct grants to the health care industry for creative ways to increase the workforce. These grants have included programs to do the following:

- Expand the pipeline of youth entering the health care profession.
- Identify alternative labor pools such as immigrants, veterans, and older workers that can be tapped and trained.
- Develop alternative training strategies for educating and training health care professionals, such as apprenticeship, distance learning, and accelerated training.
- Develop tools and curricula for enhancing the skills of health care professionals for nationwide distribution.
- Enhance the capacity of educational institutions through increased numbers of qualified faculty and new models for clinical training.
- Develop strategies to retain current health care workers and help them move into higher level positions in shortage areas.
- Help workers in declining industries build on existing skills and train for health care professions (U.S. Department of Labor, 2004).

For more information about grants directly through the Department of Labor, check their Website at (http://www.doleta.gov).

Workforce Investment Funds

The Workforce Investment Act of 1998 (WIA) was enacted to create a national workforce preparation and employment system for job seekers and employers. The goal is to develop a workforce investment system to improve the quality of the workforce, sustain economic growth, and reduce dependency on welfare (WIA, 2004). The legislation was a way to consolidate funding for programs focused on training, literacy, and vocational rehabilitation.

WIA funding is different than the former Job Training Partnership Act, which was created for the economically disadvantaged. WIA funds are much less restrictive and more geared to individual training and education by offering comprehensive career programs and tools. Services are coordinated through one-stop career centers, which provide training and employment services, including remedial educational programs. WIA funds are administered through local workforce investment boards (WIBs). WIBs include both private and public sector members, appointed by state and local officials. Examples include representatives of labor, education, community leaders, and local and state government officials. There are a variety of state agencies that distribute funds, including departments of labor and economic development. Each state, through the governor, has considerable flexibility in devising its own organizational system, membership, and funding criteria for distribution of WIA funds.

A little-known aspect of WIA funding is the opportunity to support professional education. As state workforce projects explore the opportunities for expanding the nursing workforce, one of the best potential funding sources for innovative program development is WIA funds. Mississippi, for example, has utilized WIA funds to do a study on barriers to successful completion of nursing programs and has implemented a pilot program to recruit high school students into nursing. Through the studies, funding became available to support students in undergraduate and graduate nursing educational programs. An important key for getting funding is that education must be tied into expansion of the workforce—the purpose of WIA. WIA legislation places few restrictions on funding amounts and on how funds can be used, other than that funds must be used to train people for in-demand jobs, which is defined using labor market information. Funds can be used for bachelor's degrees if local WIBs agree and there are educational institutions willing to become approved providers. Because the paperwork to become an approved provider can be cumbersome and requires educational institutions to make public some sensitive outcome data, few have been willing to become approved. However, if institutions appreciate the benefits of financial support for students and expansion of nursing programs, they can be persuaded to pursue the process of being designated as an approved provider. Often the people responsible for completing the data forms do not communicate with program administrators of recruitment and retention programs. As a result, most institutions have not appreciated the benefits of becoming approved providers. Workforce coalitions should become involved with WIB staff and determine how to lessen resistance of educational institutions to use WIA funds.

As state policy makers learn about the need to recruit people into health careers, previously untapped resources through WIA funds will likely be better utilized for preparing the nursing workforce. To accomplish this, workforce coalitions will need to be creative in developing projects and connecting them to the stipulations of WIA funding guidelines. It is also prudent to work with members of WIB to educate them about how such funds can be used for the nursing workforce. Too often, people in economic development and people in nursing workforce development have insufficient communication. Increased communication will help workforce development policy makers appreciate the positive economic impact of a qualified and adequate nursing workforce.

FOUNDATIONS

Heath Care Foundations

Foundations, especially those focused on health issues, are traditional sources of funding for nonprofit programs like state workforce projects. The impetus for the original state nursing workforce projects was the Colleagues in Caring national program, funded by the Robert Wood Johnson Foundation. Established in 1972, the Foundation is the largest philanthropy devoted exclusively to health and health care in the United States. In 2003 the Foundation changed the focus for grants, and money for the workforce projects ended. As a result, state coalitions have pursued other foundation sources, often local health foundations. Many of these have been small family-owned organizations, others have been large foundations affiliated with the health industry, such as insurance and pharmaceutical companies. Most provide public disclosure of assets and grants.

Hospital Conversion Foundations

Hospital conversion foundations were created in the mid-1980s to late 1990s when for-profit corporations were rapidly purchasing community nonprofit health institutions, such as hospitals, health systems, or health plans. To ensure a certain level of commitment to the communities, the Internal Revenue Service allowed a tax mechanism to move some of the assets from the sale of facilities to nonprofit foundations. Usually such foundations direct their funding in a limited geographic area and thus are often the largest single source of funding of health projects in a community. According to the report of Grantmakers in Health (2003), the 165 foundations identified held more than $16.5 billion in assets. Assets ranged from $1.56 million to $2.8 billion, with the average foundation assets at $46.5 million. These foundations operate in 38 states but are primarily concentrated in 10—California, Colorado, Florida, Illinois, Missouri, Ohio, Pennsylvania, North Carolina, South Carolina, and Virginia. The focus of most of their grant making is on health, human services, or other health-related activities, such as access to health care, health education, and delivery of services. Many focus on specific population groups.

The tax status of such a foundation has implications for grant making and regulatory oversight. Foundations can be defined as a private foundation, a public charity, or a social welfare organization. A significant distinction is that public charities, unlike other foundations, must also raise money from the community. Private foundations hold the largest assets and are required to make annual distributions of funds and report annually to the Internal Revenue Service.

Workforce coalitions are encouraged to discover whether such foundations exist in their state. Many of the foundations identified by Grantmakers in Health are not well known by nursing organizations and thus are not tapped for resources. Because of the urgency of the nursing shortage, such foundations, whose mission is to improve the health of their communities, should be pursued. Nursing workforce coalition leaders will need to use political skills such as advocacy, negotiation, and communication to influence foundation board members and staff to understand the connection between a strong nursing workforce and the health of communities.

A CHECKLIST FOR OBTAINING FUNDING

The first rule of funding is to have a plan. Identify the potential projects, based on a clearly defined need, and determine the resources to institute the projects. Resources are not only funds but also people, supplies, equipment, and organizational support, to name just a few. Once the coalition has developed the plan, the next step is to determine which funding sources are the most realistic to obtain. Each funding source requires a separate strategy that identifies stakeholders, political connections, and time frame. Once again, it is desirable to have different funding streams to ensure the most sustainability of projects. What follows are several basic tenets for seeking funding:

- **Know the players.** If a legislative appropriation is requested, then intensive lobbying should be focused on the policy makers who control appropriations. If foundation funding is sought, coalition members should educate staff and/or board members about the nursing shortage. Developing relationships should be a long-term strategy. Getting to know decision makers right before funding decisions are made is too late.
- **Work as a coalition of diverse groups and individuals.** This strengthens the constituency and the urgency of the funding request. Workforce coalitions should include all of the major nursing organizations in the region, as well as organizations and entities with an interest in the nursing workforce, such as departments of education, hospital representatives, and those in economic development.
- **Know the funding priorities and history of funded projects from the funding organization.** Public grant makers and foundations, in particular, define their funding priorities in their descriptive material. Find out if they ever supported workforce projects, what kinds of projects they traditionally fund, and how difficult it is to obtain funding.
- **Know how to define the relationship between workforce projects and designated funding priorities.** It often takes creativity to match the nursing project to the goals of the funder. Nontraditional sources of funding, such as workforce development funds, can yield unexpected grants if the connections are made by workforce coalitions.
- **Determine whether the amount of money is worth the effort to secure it.** Often, considerable effort is made for small

amounts of money when the same level of work could be better channeled to sources that provide large grants.

- **Stagger funding to ensure ongoing viability of the workforce entity.** If funding is staggered, workforce projects can cover periods when income is limited.

4

Gathering Nursing Workforce Data

*Linda M. Lacey, Kim Welch Hoover,
Marcella M. McKay, Eileen T. O'Grady,
and Karen Sechrist*

"He uses statistics as a drunken man uses lamp-posts . . . for support rather than illumination."

—Andrew Lang (1844–1912)

The Scottish poet, journalist, and novelist Andrew Lang inadvertently made an important point in this quotation. Statistics, and the data on which those statistics are based, can illuminate a process or phenomenon as well as support a particular position or policy. Nursing workforce planners have need for both illumination and support. A successful nursing workforce center needs accurate and reliable information about the nursing labor force and the nursing labor market in order to illuminate the trends affecting the nursing workforce and to support wise policy decisions that will affect that workforce into the future.

THE ROLE OF DATA IN A NURSING WORKFORCE CENTER

Some of the first questions that any nursing workforce center or related entity will be asked is whether there is currently a shortage of nurses, whether there will be a shortage in the future, and how many nurses are actually needed. Because the nursing labor market has suffered from cyclical shortages approximately every 10 years for the past 50 years, most observers of the phenomenon know enough to expect another one. The only real question is when. In order to answer such questions, a nursing workforce center must have a factual understanding of the supply of nurses in its area, as well as some measure of the demand for those nurses. The ways in which these two measures increase and decline in relation to each other is the basis for understanding shortage cycles. And, although the large shortages that have appeared every decade have been national in nature, not all geographic areas have been affected equally.

Another expectation of nursing workforce centers is that they be able to anticipate and/or forecast when and where the next labor shortage is likely to occur. Without accurate information collected at regular intervals, this is pretty much impossible. Even with accurate information, it is a difficult thing to do. An effective workforce center must create or have access to accurate counts of the nursing workforce (the supply side of the supply/demand equation), as well as additional information that helps to describe workforce behavior. An additional source of information is required for addressing the demand for labor that is generated from employers.

Accurate, reliable, and repeatable data bring value to a nursing workforce initiative making it worth the time, effort, and expense to secure the data. Most policy makers and legislators are reluctant to create new programs or substantially change existing policy without having some "factual" data to justify such actions. In addition to improving the decision-making process, a regular data collection and reporting schedule can also help to build understanding and support for nursing workforce issues. The Mississippi experience related later in this chapter is a good example.

IDENTIFYING DATA NEEDS RELATED TO NURSING SUPPLY

Understanding the size and composition of the nursing workforce requires timely information about the number of nurses licensed in the planning region (the potential workforce), the number of those licensed nurses who are actually employed in nursing positions (the workforce head count), and how many hours per week or per year those nurses are employed in those nursing positions (the full-time equivalent workforce). Table 4.1 contains the definition of full-time equivalent. These are the three basic measures of a labor force. The numbers generated by these measures occur at a single point in time and can be counted on to change daily. Tracking these figures

TABLE 4.1 Full-Time Equivalents

Being able to translate the number of nurses in the workforce into the actual number of full-time equivalent (FTE) positions filled within the workplace is an important refinement for workforce planners. As work patterns change, the same number of nurses might fill more or fewer full-time equivalent positions. The precision of this measure depends on the type of measure you have available for hours worked.

Decisions must also be made about what constitutes a full-time position. Ask the employers in your planning region how many hours they generally require before they consider an employee to be full time for benefit purposes. In some cases this will be 40, and in others it will be 32. Whichever you choose, make certain to report that decision in the explanation of your measure. The following examples use 40 hours per week as equal to one full-time equivalent.

1. If you have hours per week for each nurse, calculate a variable for each nurse that measures that person's FTE weight:

   FTEWT = hours per week/40

   Then sum this FTEWT field across all the nurses in your data set to arrive at a total count of FTEs in the workforce.

2. If you have only a count of the number of full-time and the number of part-time workers, then determine the FTE count for your workforce as follows:

   FTEs = total full-time workers + (total part-time workers / 2)

on a regular schedule over time allows a planner to observe changes and to use such patterns in forecasting.

In addition to the basic counts of the workforce, knowing something about each nurse's personal characteristics (e.g., age, race, gender, family structure) and about his or her work characteristics (the types of settings where the nurse is employed, the location of the employers, and the nurse's clinical specialty) can be used to refine the information about the labor force. Changes in the proportion of nurses in a single setting (e.g., a hospital) that occur over time alert workforce planners and policy makers to underlying shifts in the structure of the workplace for nurses. Similarly, demographic information can be used to understand the different factors that affect movement in and out of the workforce, and those factors then can be used to forecast the expected size and composition of the workforce in the future.

Another aspect of the supply of nurses is the capacity and rate of production in the educational pipeline that produces new nurses. How many nursing students can be admitted into prelicensure educational programs each year? How has that figure changed over time, and what factors determine the capacity of the system? Once students enter the pipeline, how many actually complete a nursing degree? Of those that complete their programs and graduate, how many actually pass the licensure exam and become eligible to enter the licensed workforce? This information, along with an understanding of how much of the total supply of new nurses is provided by the educational system in a planning region, will help planners, legislators, and policy makers know where educational resources are needed and what types of action might be appropriate during an expansion or contraction of the educational pipeline.

IDENTIFYING DATA NEEDS RELATED TO THE DEMAND FOR NURSES

Being able to accurately identify the total demand for nurses within a given planning area is virtually impossible. New roles and new opportunities are being created every day as the health care industry expands and as those outside the traditional realm of health care understand what nurses can bring to their organizations. However, it is possible to identify the traditional employment sectors that create the majority of demand for nurses within a planning region. And the largest of these organizations will collectively have the largest impact on the overall demand for nurses from one year to the next.

Measuring the demand for nurses is more complicated than measuring workforce supply. Demand is an economic concept that is affected not only by the need for nurses to fill positions but also by the wage point at which nurses are paid. *Demand* is defined as the number of nurses that employers are willing to hire at a specific wage point. As wages rise, the demand for nurses may be reduced. As wages decrease, the number of nurses that employers can afford to hire increases. Wages matter in the determination of demand for nurses. However, few measures of demand incorporate wage levels into the question. One of the most common ways in which future demand is estimated is by asking employers to report the total number of budgeted positions currently existing and then to predict how many budgeted positions will be added or subtracted in the coming year or in the next two or three years. This type of question format is relatively easy for respondents to answer but makes the silent assumption that wage levels will not change to a meaningful degree. This type of demand measure also results in a count of new job openings for nurses but does not include the need for replacements for nurses who leave the profession due to retirement, death, burnout, or other reason.

One of the most commonly seen statistics is one that is presented as a measure of demand, but actually is a measure of the imbalance between supply and demand—vacancy rate. There are two different measures of vacancy, one that provides an average of facility-level data that reports the percentage of budgeted positions that are vacant and being recruited at a specific point in time (average vacancy rate) and another that summarizes all vacant positions over a planning area and reports the total percentage of positions that are vacant and being recruited (position vacancy rate) (see Table 4.2). Both measurement approaches are useful but provide different views of the balance of supply and demand in a planning region. The one most often reported is an average of the facility-level measure. So, for example, consider the statement that State ABC has a 12.5% vacancy rate. Chances are what this really means is that the average vacancy rate across all facilities responding to that study was 12.5%. That statistic does not specify whether there were facilities with either very high or very low vacancy rates that might be affecting that value.

The average vacancy rate is actually a very useful planning tool inasmuch as it requires that each facility be measured individually. (When comparing data from different entities to one another, it is best if the raw elements that make up the measure be collected and then the final product calculated by the researcher. This ensures that the same concept is being measured in a consistent manner.) From a planning perspective, one of the most difficult situations to define is whether a true labor shortage exists (i.e., too few nurses in the aggregate to fill the total number of positions being recruited) or whether simply a number of facilities are having difficulty recruiting and/or retaining an adequate number of nurses and are thus influencing the findings. Knowing the distribution of vacancy rates across all employers in the planning region makes it possible to answer this question. And although there is no official definition of how high vacancy rates must be across some percentage of employers in order to signal a true shortage, experience and repeated measures over time will tell planners whether things are getting better or worse in their region or for that sector of employers. Facility-level vacancy rates can also point out which employers or which employment sectors (i.e., hospitals, long-term care, home health, etc.) are

TABLE 4.2   Nursing Workforce Measure: Vacancy Rate

A *position vacancy rate* provides a rate based on the total number of available positions for a specific type of employee within a specific region or industry. It aggregates the number of positions (vacant plus filled) over all employing organizations in a planning region or within an industry grouping (e.g., hospitals), and provides the percentage of those total positions that are not currently filled. It can also be interpreted in terms of absolute numbers of employees needed in that region or industry. The calculation is as follows:

Position vacancy rate =
(total # of vacant positions / (total vacant positions + total filled
    positions)) x 100

Example: Hospital A has 100 filled FTE positions for RNs and 5 unfilled ones. Hospital B has 50 filled FTEs for RNs and 5 unfilled ones. Hospital C has 25 filled positions and 5 unfilled ones.

$$((5 + 5 + 5) / ((5 + 5 + 5) + (100 + 50 + 25)) = 15 / (15 + 175) =$$
$$0.789 \times 100 = 7.89\%$$

An *average vacancy rate,* on the other hand, creates the vacancy rate within each employing organization and then averages that information over all the participating organizations. The result can be very different from the value created by the position vacancy rate method. An average rate gives each organization equal weight in the calculation regardless of the size of the organization or the total number of positions that are vacant. The calculation for an average vacancy rate is as follows:

Average vacancy rate =
((SUM (vacant positions in each agency / (vacant + filled positions in
    each agency)) / total number of participating agencies) x 100

Example: Using the same example cases presented above:

$$(((5/100) + (5/50) + (5/25)) / 3) = ((0.05 + 0.10 + 0.20) / 3) =$$
$$0.11666 \times 100 = 11.67\%$$

doing relatively well or poorly in terms of their ability to attract the workforce they need. Having a few facilities with very high vacancy rates while the remainder have low rates is most likely an indication that wage rates in those facilities are substantially lower than in the rest of the market, or that there are other factors within those organizational environments that make them undesirable for nurses.

Another statistic often presented as evidence of shortage is the turnover rate, which is the percentage of employees (whether RNs, LPNs, nurse aides, new hires, etc.) that leave an organization during some specific period of time, usually annually (see Table 4.3). This is a measure that can only occur at the facility level and is, in fact, only an indication of how well or how poorly a specific employer retains those kinds of employees. Turnover from one employer to another has no effect on the overall size of the workforce and thus does not affect overall demand or supply.

STATE-LEVEL DATA SOURCES

Few nursing workforce centers have the time, money, or qualified staff to conduct the types of demand studies that can produce accurate counts of the number of nurses needed at a specific point in time for an entire region. Luckily, most states do have an agency of state government that can do this type of work. Under different names and different sections of government, these agencies may be able to provide demand estimates for planners or consultation services to nursing workforce centers that want to develop their own data system. Although not focused on nursing specifically, these agencies conduct annual surveys of industries and employers to measure the number of new jobs employers expect to create. This information is organized along occupational lines and shared with the Bureau of Labor Statistics (BLS). They, in turn, use employment patterns data from multiple national surveys such as the Current Population Survey and Occupational Employment Survey to forecast the number of replacements that will be needed in each occupation as people retire, die, or leave that occupational workforce for other reasons. Together these data sources form the basis of the national-level BLS Occupational Outlook series of reports which aggregates all state-level data together.

State agencies involved with workforce issues in general are a good place to start when seeking information about either supply or demand issues. The Department of Commerce, workforce development boards, and the agency that administers unemployment benefits will all have knowledge about where such information can be found in your state. Because these agencies have a broader focus than just one professional group, it may be necessary to develop a working relationship with them over time in order to get what you need. And even if they don't have the type of data that you seek, they probably have someone on staff with the type of expertise you need to design a workable data collection strategy.

Supply data related to licensees may be found in most state Boards of Nursing, along with information about the size and shape

TABLE 4.3   Nursing Workforce Measure: Turnover Rate

Turnover rates should always be calculated only on those employees who have been formally on the payroll for at least one pay period and who have left the organization. Do not count employees who transfer to another position within the organization. Only those actually lost to the organization should be included in this measure. This measure is a count of people rather than positions. Thus, if multiple individuals filled one position during the period being studied, each one should be counted in the numerator.

The definitional equation that follows uses an annual study period (2003). Any time period can be used, as long as both the numerator and denominator use the same time period.

Turnover rate = (total number of employees who left the organization between 1/1/2003 and 12/31/2003) / ((number of employees as of 1/1/2003 + number of employees as of 12/31/2003) / 2) x 100

of the educational pipeline if that agency has regulatory authority over pre-licensure education. Some states have "super" boards that combine multiple regulatory agencies under one administrative umbrella. These agencies may have data related to nurses, or may be the appropriate agency to negotiate with to see that such data is collected in the future. If your state has no formal data collection effort underway for nursing, it may be possible to find enough data to approximate your basic supply measures from national studies and surveys.

REGIONAL AND NATIONAL DATA SOURCES

In addition to state-level sources of information there are regional and national sources that might provide either supply-side or demand-side data that can be used for some aspects of workforce planning.

Bureau of Health Professions/Health Resources and Services Administration

The national Bureau of Health Professions, located within the Health Resources and Services Administration (HRSA), supports six regional centers for health workforce studies across the country that examine issues involving cross-disciplinary assessments of the health workforce at the state and regional levels. Specific projects vary by regional center, but each is directly involved in measuring and assessing the adequacy of the health professions in their regions, including nursing. As of 2004 six regional centers had been funded. Center-specific information can be obtained from the Bureau of Health Professions website at http://bhpr.hrsa.gov/healthworkforce/centers/default.htm

HRSA and the Bureau of Health Professions also maintains two public use database files developed from each of the National Sample Survey of Registered Nurses which are conducted approximately every four years. The General Public Use file provides survey responses at the state level and includes educational attainment, employment status, income and other demographic information from survey respondents. The County Public Use file provides additional geographic fields for Metropolitan Statistical Area and county level identification. Fields that could identify the respondent are withheld to protect privacy. Each response has a statistical sampling weight, allowing the user to make workforce estimates. The largest and most recent database is the 2000 survey, with more than 35,000 respondents. Other available years are: 1977, 1980, 1984, 1988, 1992, 1996.

In states that have little or no information about their nursing workforce, this data source can provide a beginning point for workforce profiles. Analysis of specialty groups within nursing such as nurse practitioners or nurse midwives becomes problematic at the state level with this data because the sampling frame was not designed for such purposes and the actual number of respondents in a particular state may be too small to support reliable analysis.

In addition, HRSA and the Bureau of Health Professions have developed nursing supply and demand forecasting models that provide state-level estimates. Older versions of these models were difficult to use, but newer models have been developed in recent years that allow states to estimate future RN supply figures at different levels of analysis (i.e., total licensed population, total workforce head counts, and estimated full-time equivalent workforce) and to estimate future demand projections for both RNs and LPNs/LVNs (along with nurse aides and home health aides), given the economic conditions, population needs, and the health care operating environment with the state. The models are constructed so that baseline data intrinsic to the models may be used, or states can substitute their own baseline numbers to generate the forecasts.

Bureau of Labor Statistics/U.S. Department of Labor

The federal Bureau of Labor Statistics (BLS) also creates future forecasts of demand for RNs, LPNs/LVNs, and nurse aides—both at the national and the state level. Easily accessible through their web site, the Office of Occupational Statistics and Employment Projections at the BLS reports both current employment (i.e., demand) levels and forecasts expected demand 10 years into the future. These demand projections, updated every two years, include two different aspects of demand: new job growth and replacement openings caused by death, retirement, disability or career changes. Being able to see these two different aspects of demand for nurses is a valuable asset for workforce planners. One of the disadvantages of this data source is that the RN figures reported by BLS are primarily direct-care nurses, since nurses in management, administration, and educational positions are included in those occupational categories, rather than under the registered nurse code. In addition, advanced practice nurses are not classified separately from other direct-care nurses. The negative effect of this is probably most influential in the salary data reported by BLS, since NP and CRNA salaries are significantly higher than most other nurses and will skew the data. But this shortcoming should not preclude an examination of BLS databases. To determine if BLS data might be useful for local planning efforts, conduct a retroactive examination of the numbers BLS has produced in their biennial projections of employment and occupations to see how well (or poorly) their numbers agree with what you know to be true in your area.

Other National Data Sources

The Interagency Conference on Nursing Statistics (ICONS) is an informal voluntary association representing a wide variety of nursing organizations that collect or have collected nursing data. ICONS' objective is to promote the generation and utilization of data, information, and research to facilitate decisions about nurses, nursing education, and the workforce by using existing sources of data. ICONS does not directly conduct research, but does monitor available data sources. Contact them to inquire about what types of data might be available and appropriate for state-level planning purposes.

National nursing organizations and associations may also be sources of data. The National League for Nursing, the American Association of Colleges of Nursing, the American Nurses Association, the National Council of State Boards of Nursing, and associations devoted to clinical specialty areas within nursing such as the American Academy of Nurse Practitioners and others may have information and/or data sources that can be used in your planning efforts. The California Strategic Planning Model profiled later in this chapter is a good example of how several different secondary sources of data can be combined to create an ongoing profile of the nursing workforce.

PRIMARY DATA COLLECTION

Of course, there is always the option of collecting the data directly. But regardless of who does the data collection, the information is only as good as the instrument used to collect it, and any results generated are only as good as the data that went into the analysis. Garbage in, garbage out, as researchers say.

One of the guiding principles of many researchers and most data managers is that you should only collect the data that you will need to answer your research question. Collecting data from scratch, organizing the data, and analyzing the results can be difficult and expensive and, as such, should not be taken on lightly. Primary data collection is a multifaceted task. It involves clearly defining the research or administrative questions to be answered; translating those questions into operational definitions so that specific concepts can be identified; locating (or developing) accurate and appropriate measures of those concepts; creating a survey question, or series of questions, that can be answered accurately and reliably by the person completing the survey; developing a survey tool that is easy to read and understand and is not so long that it negatively affects response rates; developing a survey strategy that will ensure that the resulting data are representative and can be extrapolated to the entire population of nurses in the planning region; ensuring that the sampling strategy will result in enough cases to make statistical analysis possible and reliable; and developing and implementing a strategy to ensure an adequate response rate.

Then, after you have decided on how to administer your survey (mailed questionnaire, telephone survey, Internet survey, etc.), you must devote the appropriate resources to getting it done in a timely manner. The way in which survey responses will be entered into a database will depend on how the survey is administered. Regardless, accuracy is of prime importance.

Finally, once the data are available for analysis in raw form, each data point needs to be checked for accuracy, cleaned to remove obvious errors, and put into a format that will allow the type of analysis that is dictated by the questions you want answered and the level of measurement in your data. An experienced analyst should be brought in to provide consultation or to complete the statistical analysis, if possible. Knowing which statistics can be used with which types of data and how to interpret the results correctly is a specialized skill. Even with impeccable data, without the proper skills the data analyst can make many mistakes when interpreting what the data patterns actually mean.

Clearly, primary data collection is not a job for the fainthearted or ill prepared. However, sometimes it is the only option. When done well, the information and new knowledge created will be useful not only to workforce planners but also to nurse employers, nursing educators, nurses, legislators, and others. Thus, one of the benefits of generating new data can be an opportunity to build support coalitions between your nursing workforce center or initiative and other stakeholder organizations that are interested in the information you have developed. Although all data should be treated as confidential to protect the respondents, sharing data in an aggregated form or with identifiers stripped off is a practice that can help generate support or even funding for your organization. Developing a data system with a reputation for accuracy and reliability can contribute to the sustainability of your nursing workforce center. Mississippi's experience is a good example: Coalitions contributed to the collection of quality data, and coalitions resulted from sharing that data.

BUILDING A STANDARDIZED DATABASE FOR NURSING WORKFORCE ISSUES

One of the goals that grew out of the Colleagues in Caring (CIC) project was the development of a standard data set that can serve the needs of nursing workforce centers across the country. Once in place and in use by all states, such a standardized data set could also be used to make state-to-state comparisons, aggregated into multistate planning regions, allow regional analysis of nursing workforce issues, and provide the basis for an unduplicated count of the nursing workforce across the United States.

During the last two years of the CIC project, a standardized data set (see appendix A) was defined for the nursing supply. It was developed specifically as a minimum data template, the idea being that each state needs each of the identified pieces of information, at minimum, to do a proper job of workforce analysis. The data set contains 13 questions and 33 data fields. The answer categories were designed to be the minimum necessary and can be expanded to meet the needs of a particular planning region, as long as any expansion categories can be aggregated back into the original categories. Of course, if resources allow, additional questions can also be added. But the idea behind the minimum supply data set was to keep the cost and complexity of data collection at a minimum. Usually implemented as part of the license renewal process in conjunction with the state board of nursing, the Minimum Supply Data Set template has already been adopted by several states. However, many states still struggle with inadequate funding and limited resources that place data collection, however minimal, far down the list of priorities.

Perhaps the best chance for creating a standardized database of information about the supply of nurses in this country is to involve the National Council of State Boards of Nursing (NCSBN) in a central role. This national organization is the umbrella association for the separate state regulatory boards of nursing. As such, it has taken positive steps toward promoting uniformity in the regulation of nursing practice, disseminating information related to the licensure of nurses, conducting research pertinent to their purpose, and serving as a forum for information exchange among members. Their values include "forging solutions through the collective strength of internal and external stakeholders" (NCSBN, 2004). Given its orientation toward the future and its appreciation for the importance of quality data in addressing nursing workforce issues, NCSBN seems like a natural partner for nursing workforce centers and their constituent boards of nursing. The NCSBN has experience in developing a centralized database made from data contributions from state boards. Its Nurse Information System has become an invaluable resource for both nurse employers and state boards of nursing. If NCSBN adopted the Minimum Supply Data Set template and data field definitions as its standard for workforce data, a truly national database could be developed relatively quickly. As more and more state boards of nursing turn to online license renewal, the capture of those data could also be standardized, centralized, and possibly even sent directly to NCSBN. And although not all states are currently using online technology for license renewal, the cost savings over paper forms will soon make online renewal the technology of choice. In states that are already online, approximately 75%–85% of nurses are using electronic renewal options (P. Johnson, personal communication, June 2004).

State Nursing Workforce Data:
California and Mississippi

The following exemplars provide a glimpse into the many ways that data are gathered and used to create knowledge about a state's nursing workforce. The end results are similar, but the pathways followed by these workforce planners were different.

The California Strategic Nursing Planning Model

The California Strategic Planning Committee for Nursing (CSPCN) was formed in December 1992 by nurse leaders in response to a need for reliable data for public policy and resource allocation decisions to meet California's need for nurses. Based on group consensus that a master planning process for RNs and LVNs needed to be initiated and maintained in the state, CSPCN began the California Nursing Workforce Initiative in January 1994. Objectives for the initiative were to (1) develop and maintain a dynamic forecasting model to predict the nursing workforce California's people would need for their health care, (2) develop a strategic plan to ensure the supply of nurses meets the demand, and (3) implement the plan.

Development of a forecast modeling process to project demand for and supply of nursing personnel was the first task. One of the problems in developing a model was the fact that many forecasting methods, by design, reflect expectations that future events will follow previous patterns. This assumption was considered invalid in the climate of downsizing, changes in location of health care delivery services, and organizational mergers that were occurring in the health care industry at the time. Further, many forecasting approaches were expensive and labor-intensive. Cost-effectiveness, relative ease of data collection, and sensitivity to changing patterns were deemed to be desirable hallmarks of a nursing workforce forecasting process.

A multimethod approach to determining nurse demand and supply evolved because no single mechanism provided the expectations of success. Key considerations in selection of methodologies were the balancing of (1) historical trend data with the impact of changing patterns, (2) level of accuracy with cost constraints, (3) use of available data with costs of collecting additional data, and (4) time required to obtain data with the urgency of current need for projections.

CSPCN's Strategic Planning Model is shown in Figure 4.1. The Nurse Demand and Nurse Supply components of the Model are composed of existing and project-specific data elements that have

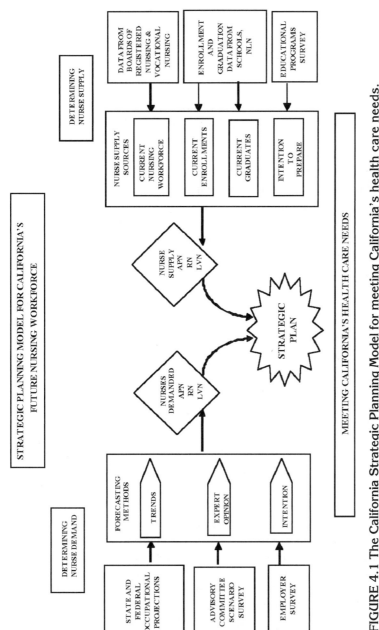

FIGURE 4.1 The California Strategic Planning Model for meeting California's health care needs.

Reprinted with permission of the California Strategic Committee for Nursing (Project Office: University of California, Irvine College of Medicine, Bldg 802, Room 290, Irvine, CA 92697-4089). © CSPN, 1995.

proved useful in gaining insight into nurse demand and nurse supply for the purpose of strategic planning. An assessment of the adequacy of the nursing workforce and strategic recommendations are derived from a synthesis of the components.

Demand for Nursing Personnel. Insight into the demand for nursing personnel in California was obtained using three approaches. First, existing state and federal occupational projections were reviewed. These macrolevel models project general occupational growth for RNs and LVNs. Second, scenarios within which health care is likely to occur were summarized from expert opinion literature, surveys, and conference reports. Third, data concerning the intention of health care providers to employ nursing personnel were obtained through an employer sample survey. The responses about employment patterns for various types of nursing personnel in a current year and intended employment of nursing personnel over the subsequent three-year period provided information on trends in demand for varying types of registered nurses across multiple health care delivery sectors.

Nurse Supply. Four categories of information were used to determine nurse supply. Information on the current nursing workforce was obtained from several sources. The numbers of nurses holding active licenses to practice nursing in California as an RN or LVN were obtained from the California Board of Registered Nursing (BRN) and the California Board of Vocational Nurses and Psychiatric Technicians (BVNPT). Demographic and practice characteristics of California RNs were summarized from three sources: (1) sample survey data files of RNs with active California licenses conducted by the BRN, (2) the Nurse Information System (NIS) survey data file of RNs applying for relicensure conducted by the NCBSN in collaboration with the BRN, and (3) the California sample data file from the National Sample Survey of Registered Nurses (NSS) conducted by the Department of Health and Human Services, Division of Nursing. Information about current enrollments in prelicensure nursing programs was obtained from the BRN, the National League for Nursing (NLN), and the American Association of Colleges of Nursing (AACN). Likewise, information on current graduates was obtained from the BRN, NLN, and AACN. Information on the intention to enroll students in programs of nursing leading to LVN and RN licensure, advanced practice preparation, and graduate degrees was obtained initially from nursing education program administrators. These data are now included in the annual enrollment and graduation report for the BRN.

Data were collected and synthesized into reports three times between 1994 and 2003 (Sechrist & Lewis, 1996; Sechrist, Lewis, & Rutledge, 1999; Sechrist, Lewis, Rutledge, & Keating, 2002). The three reports identified the need for increased numbers of RNs and LVNs in general and the specific need for increased numbers of RNs with bachelor's and master's degrees. These needs were identified even during the period of hospital downsizing in the mid-1990s. The reports were used by nurse leaders to advocate for increased support for nursing education.

Mississippi's Story: Lessons Learned for Facilitating Data Collection

"Small opportunities are often the beginnings of great enterprises."
—Demosthenes (384–322 BC)

Mississippians have often been described as the consummate deal makers with their tendency to agree on issues of extreme importance over lunch or a cup of coffee. Often, a handshake and someone's word seal the deal. The story of Mississippi's successful workforce data collection and influence has been shared in numerous venues by the authors and others such as Peggy O. Hewlett, PhD, RN, past director of the Mississippi Office of Nursing Workforce (MONW) and current associate dean of research at the University of Mississippi Medical Center School of Nursing (UMMC SON); Judith K. Leavitt, MEd, RN, FAAN, current chair of MONW Advisory Committee and associate professor at UMMC SON; Wanda Jones, MSN, RN, current executive director of MONW; and Betty Dickson, executive director of the Mississippi Nurses Association (MNA). This section describes development of the data collection process and the lessons learned.

One cannot begin to understand the benefits of data collection and nursing workforce relationships in Mississippi without a brief history of the Mississippi Office of Nursing Workforce (MONW), for therein lie the simplicities and complexities of MONW data collection and influence. In 1994 and 1995, nursing leaders in Mississippi recognized that although nursing organizations individually had worthy goals and issues, the organizations together could affect nursing problems more effectively by speaking with one collective voice. Consequently, a dormant Mississippi Nurses Association (MNA) committee known as the Nursing Organization Liaison Committee (NOLC) was revived, and representatives from 25 nursing organizations across the state began to focus on the impact of the changing health care environment on nursing in Mississippi.

At that time, managed care had resulted in sweeping changes across the nation and nursing leaders were interested in identifying and equipping nurses with new skills that might be needed for the future, such as case management. The prevailing thought was to examine statewide needs rather than local or regional needs. Discussions focused on how health care reform had affected health care and nursing in Mississippi and how nursing leaders might better equip themselves to more fully integrate nurses into future health care changes. Inevitably, the group focused on the need for valid and reliable data upon which to base decisions regarding current and future needs.

The group recognized that a projected comprehensive nursing data system was beyond the scope of one organization and would require cooperative effort and substantial funding. Ultimately, two major funding sources were pursued simultaneously, the Robert Wood Johnson Foundation CIC grant and Mississippi legislative funding. Through the efforts of NOLC, the Mississippi legislature passed the Nursing Workforce Redevelopment Act during the 1996 session to authorize the board of nursing to establish an entity to address changes impacting the nursing workforce and appropriated $100,000 for the 1996 fiscal year. The grant-writing team was also successful in obtaining the CIC grant. The leaders of the initiative examined the legislative language and the CIC grant objectives and decided to combine the efforts, once again making the decision that the collective voice was stronger than the individual voice. The Mississippi Office of Nursing Workforce Redevelopment was established, and Dr. Hewlett became the first project director.

The original grant-writing group was a unique cluster composed of nurses and others who held influential positions in state entities such as the MNA, the Mississippi State Department of Health (MSDH), the Mississippi Hospital Association (MHA), and the Mississippi Council of Deans and Directors of Schools of Nursing. The majority of this group would eventually serve as the original advisory committee for MONW. Those who helped establish the office had the respect and trust of the health care community and political clout within the state as a whole. The legislature was convinced that MONW was a worthwhile endeavor and had bought in. Already, the influence of the newly created office was destined to have an impact on more than the nursing area and to have the support of more than nursing organizations. The importance of relationships became increasingly evident as MONW evolved and the office was sustained beyond the end of Robert Wood Johnson Foundation funding cycles.

The advisory committee for MONW realized that data were crucial to help drive decision making for nursing and health care in the future, even if the "honeymoon" phase of influence enjoyed by the newly created office did not last. At the same time, CIC groups across the United States were networking and model data systems were being developed. Consultants were identified to assist in actualizing MONW's legislative mandate and CIC goals. Dr. Karen Sechrist from California was hired as a consultant to assist in the development of a data collection tool. Mississippi's data collection tool was modeled after California's nursing workforce data survey, described earlier in this chapter, and although this tool has undergone several revisions, it remains quite similar in content and structure.

This is where Mississippi's data collection story becomes unique. In an effort to save scarce dollars and to ensure a high return rate, MONW worked through a partnership with the Mississippi Department of Health Division of Licensure and Certification to send the nursing workforce surveys as an addendum to facility licensure renewal forms. The initial surveys went to all licensed health care facilities, including hospitals, long-term care facilities, and home health agencies. These health care facilities employ 75% of registered nurses working full or part time in nursing in the state (Mississippi Board of Nursing, 2003). This was possible, in part, because an original grant writer and advisory committee member, Dr. Kaye Bender, held the second highest position within the MSDH and was willing to facilitate communication between MSDH and MONW staff. The survey and a cover letter were printed by MONW and placed in the same envelope as the licensure and certification documents with instructions to complete and return the data forms with the licensure documents. This strategy worked well, particularly with long-term care facilities. While the surveys were voluntary, and still are, many facilities were motivated to return the survey because it was attached to regulatory forms.

Hospitals responded well, but because these entities were the largest employer of nurses in the state of Mississippi, MONW wanted responses from hospitals employing the greatest number of nurses. Since the Mississippi Hospital Association (MHA) Health, Research and Education Foundation was serving as the fiduciary agency for MONW, the Foundation's chief executive, Dr. Marcella McKay, personally contacted chief nursing officers and/or chief executives of nonresponding hospitals and solicited their input. Recognizing the competitive nature of hospital leaders, she encouraged nonresponding hospitals to send data to ensure their hospital's data were included in regional data used for public policy decision making because other hospitals in their area had already returned nursing workforce surveys. As a result of creative surveying and vigilant tactics, Mississippi achieved an astounding 75%–90% annual return rate from both hospitals and long-term care facilities. As the survey became established as an annual data collection, MONW reported data annually to the legislature, in the Mississippi State Health Plan, and as a service to public and private organizations with data needs. As the role of MONW and the value of annual nursing data were recognized by health care organizations and the public, annual response rates improved. Long-term care facilities typically respond at a 75%–85% rate, and in 2004 MONW achieved an extraordinary 96% response rate for hospitals.

MONW has enjoyed an ongoing positive relationship with the Mississippi Board of Nursing (MBON). MONW was created under the auspices of the MBON, the executive director is an ex officio member of the MONW advisory committee, and the MBON has consistently provided access to a full range of nursing supply data. Additionally, the Mississippi Council of Deans and Directors of Schools of Nursing lent their support by agreeing to help develop and participate in a survey of schools of nursing regarding faculty and students.

In addition to statewide relationships, national collaborative partnerships were cultivated. The most obvious relationships have been with the other CIC projects, such as those in California, North Carolina, and Arizona. One example of a recent national collaboration was with the Southern Regional Education Board Council on Collegiate Education for Nursing (SREB). Historically, in Mississippi, the board of trustees of Institutions of Higher Learning (IHL), the state accrediting body for schools of nursing, required the deans and directors of schools of nursing to complete a mandatory survey with data similar to data solicited by MONW. Not only was there duplication of data, but the forms required by IHL were not user friendly and typically were frustrating to complete. Data gleaned from the forms were often inaccurate. MONW also had a nursing program survey that was lengthy and somewhat duplicative.

In 2002, SREB implemented a survey to elicit information on enrollment, reasons for not admitting students, and faculty issues (e.g., retirement), within their membership of 16 states and the District of Columbia. A review of the survey indicated that it was more comprehensive than the MONW or the IHL surveys. After receiving the approval of the Deans and Directors Council, the chief executive, Dr. Eula Aiken, was contacted to negotiate a mutually beneficial method of surveying schools of nursing in Mississippi.

SREB sent the surveys, but they were routed through MONW for copying before the originals were returned to SREB. In return, MONW encouraged participation in the survey. Mississippi was the only state surveyed that had 100% participation by schools of nursing. Through this partnership, MONW provided accurate strategic planning data for the schools and avoided duplication of surveys while expanding existing databases.

Mississippi's story for data collection and analysis obviously is a continuing one. However, the data have been used to advance a public policy agenda for continuing to fund the MONW in tight budgetary times. This story is continued in chapter 7.

5

Redesign of Nursing Work

Donna Sullivan Havens, Edna Cadmus, Karen S. Cox, Jill Fuller, and Susan Lacey

"It is timely to consider a thoughtful discourse on the present shortage, which is more sustained than any other, as the future is shaped."

—Ferguson, 1990

An important element among strategic solutions for ensuring an optimal nursing workforce is a focus on the work environment for nurses. A conceptual introduction to work redesign is followed by specific exemplars in this chapter.

THE NEED TO REDESIGN NURSING WORK

When nurses were asked how they felt when they left work each day, the four most frequent responses were "exhausted and discouraged"; "discouraged and saddened by what I couldn't provide for my patients"; "powerless to affect change necessary for safe, quality patient care"; and "frightened for patients" (Brown, 2002). Most of the nurses (83%) responding to the survey reported that the solution to the current cyclical nursing shortage is to "improve the working environment." In a five-country study, more than 41% of U.S. nurses reported being dissatisfied with their jobs (Aiken, Clarke, Sloane, Sochalsky, Busse, et al., 2001). It is even more alarming that 54% of U.S. nurses reported burnout scores in the "high" range—more than nurses from any of the other participating countries (Aiken, Clarke, & Sloane, 2002). Research has shown that these conditions are associated with the work environment, that they impact both patient and nurse outcomes, and that they have contributed to recurrent nurse shortages over past decades.

Decades of research have consistently pointed to the same needed approaches to stem these problems—strategies to improve the working environment to enhance the quality of work life and the quality of care. Thus, after more than 20 years of calls to attenuate these problems, the following remains relevant: "One of the greatest needs of our time, so often disregarded, is to capture that which works and replicate it when it suits" (Ferguson, 1983).

THE RELATIONSHIP BETWEEN NURSING WORK ENVIRONMENTS AND OUTCOMES

Research has demonstrated that the way nurses are organized affects the quality of the working environment and nurse, patient, and organizational outcomes. For instance, organizational attributes that are features of professional nursing practice models, such as participative management, decentralized administration, supportive administration, and a high degree of nurse-physician collaboration, have been associated with greater nurse satisfaction (Aiken, Havens, & Sloane, 2000; Blegen, 1993; Jones, 1996; Langemo, Anderson, & Volden, 2002; Laschinger & Havens, 1996a, 1996b, 1997; Laschinger, Shamian, & Thomson, 2001; Leveck & Jones, 1996; Mark, Salyer, & Wan, 2003); greater intent to stay (Baggs, Schmitt, Mushlin, Eldredge, Oakes, & Hutson, 1997; Davidson, Folcarelli, Crawford, Duprat, & Clifford, 1997; Hinshaw, Smeltzer, & Atwood, 1987; Leveck & Jones, 1996; Taunton, Boyle, Woods, Hansen, & Bott, 1997); less job strain and burnout (Aiken, Havens, & Sloane, 2000; Davidson et al., 1997; deJonge, Bosma, Peter, & Siegrist, 2000; Kalliath & Beck, 2001; Laschinger & Havens, 1996a, 1996b, 1997; Laschinger, Shamian, & Thomson, 2001); and fewer psychosomatic and physical complaints and documented physical disorders (deJonge, Bosma, Peter, & Siegrist, 2000; Elsass & Veiga, 1997; Karasek & Theorell, 1990). In addition, nurses working in hospitals with weak organizational support for nursing care were twice as likely to report dissatisfaction and high levels of burnout (Aiken, Havens, & Sloane, 2000).

The features of the work environment have also been associated with patient outcomes, including higher nurse-reported quality of care (Aiken, Havens, & Sloane, 2000; Cassard, Weisman, Gordon, & Wong, 1994; Havens, 2001; Karasek & Theorell, 1990; Leveck & Jones, 1996); lower patient mortality and fewer complications (Aiken, Smith, & Lake, 1994; Baggs, Schmitt, Muschlin, Eldredge, Oakes, & Hutson, 1997; Knaus, Draper, Wagner, & Zimmerman,

1986; Mitchell, Armstrong, Simpson, & Lentz, 1989); shorter mean length of stay (Aiken, Clarke, et al., 1999); less use of ICU days (Aiken, Sloane, et al., 1999); and more satisfaction with pain medication (Wild & Mitchell, 2000).

Finally, features of professional practice environments have also been empirically linked with organizational outcomes such as lower nurse turnover (Hinshaw, Smeltzer, & Atwood, 1987; Leveck & Jones, 1996; Lucas, Atwood, & Hagaman, 1993; Mark, Salyer, & Wan, 2003); organizational turnover costs (Jones, 1990a, 1990b), and greater organizational commitment (Corey-Lisle, Tarzian, Cohen, & Trinkoff, 1999). In addition, the links between satisfaction and retention are well established in the literature (Blegen, 1993; Boyle, Bott, Hansen, Woods, & Taunton, 1999; Davidson et al., 1997; Leveck & Jones, 1996; Price & Mueller, 1981; Seago, Ash, Spetz, Coffman, & Grumbach, 2001).

Clearly, research suggests associations between the way nurses are organized-the design of nursing work—and the quality of the working environment and patient and nurse outcomes. In other words, healthy work environments promote healthy patients and staff (Eisenberg, Bowman, & Foster, 2001).

BUILDING WORK ENVIRONMENTS THAT WORK

The nursing shortage of the late 1970s prompted the creation of several task forces and at least four principal national studies to explore what was dissatisfying about nursing work (Institute of Medicine, 1983; American Hospital Association, 1983; U.S. Department of Health and Human Services, 1988; Veteran's Administration Health Care Amendments of 1980). Based on the findings of these studies, more than 70 recommendations emerged. All the reports called for significant micro- and macro-level changes in the organization of nursing work to increase the attractiveness of the profession as a career. Likewise, Jacox (1982) called for "serious reconstruction of the hospital nurse's role to make more efficient and effective use of nurses' knowledge and abilities" (p. 89). She identified three overlapping areas in need of attention: (1) the work of nursing itself, (2) the working conditions, and (3) the relationship of the nurse to the total hospital organization.

At the same time, another national study was conducted by the American Academy of Nursing (AAN), the magnet hospital study (McClure, Poulin, Sovie, & Wandelt, 1983). The magnet study came from a different perspective from that of most others. The purposes of the magnet study were to determine what nurses found satisfying about their work and working environments and to identify the features found in hospitals that were known as excellent places for nurses to work and for patients to receive care so that others could learn and implement these features into the organization of nursing practice to improve care and nurse well-being.

In the late 1990s and early 2000s, concerns once again surfaced about nurse workforce shortages, working conditions, and patient safety. In response, the Agency for Healthcare Research and Quality (AHRQ), National Institute for Occupational Safety and Health (NIOSH), Occupational Safety and Health Administration (OSHA), and the Veterans Health Administration (VHA) collaborated to sponsor two conferences: The Effect of Working Conditions on the Quality of Care in 1999 and Enhancing Working Conditions and Patient Safety: Best Practices in 2000. These meetings were designed to close the gaps between what is known and what needs to be known about the association between working conditions and a specific aspect of quality and patient safety (Eisenberg, Bowman, & Foster, 2001). The proceedings from the two conferences suggested that certain key workplace factors influence the quality of care because they affected the workplace and therefore affected workers. The conference reports called for the creation of healthy work environments "where workers will be able to deliver higher quality care and in which worker health and patient care quality are mutually supportive" (Eisenberg et al., 2001, p. 447). According to Eisenberg et al., (2001) in the healthy workplace model, "the physical and emotional health of workers fosters quality care, and vice versa, being able to deliver high-quality care fosters worker health" (p. 447). In other words, the quality of the work environment influences the quality of the work, which influences the quality of outcomes for workers and patients.

Although there is a growing body of literature to substantiate that health care workers experience work environment stressors associated with strain, job dissatisfaction, burnout, intentions to quit, and reduced mental health, there is also evidence that work redesign interventions can be implemented to attenuate these conditions. For instance, according to Sainfort, Karsh, Booske, and Smith (2001), workplace interventions can be designed to improve organizational effectiveness and decrease employee stress by manipulating variables such as

- management practices (e.g., improvement programs, career development, strategic planning, human resources planning, and fair pay and rewards)

- organizational climate (e.g., innovation, cooperation, diversity, conflict resolution, and sense of belonging)
- organizational values (e.g., employee growth and development and valuing the individual worker)

The magnet hospital model is a long-standing and popular "best practice" organizational exemplar that has been associated with excellent nursing work environments and excellent patient care (Aiken, Havens, & Sloane, 2000; Havens, 2001; Havens & Aiken, 1999; McClure & Hinshaw, 2002). Magnet organizations are characterized by high levels of nurse autonomy, control, and collaboration with physicians (Havens & Aiken, 1999; McClure & Hinshaw, 2002; McClure, Poulin, Sovie, & Wandelt, 1983). Furthermore, the magnet principles bear a close resemblance to the principles suggested by Sainfort, Karsh, Booske, and Smith (2001) to promote healthy work environments.

Magnet Hospital Principles

Since 1982, two groups of hospitals have been designated as magnet hospitals: (1) the original magnets, selected in 1982 by American Academy of Nursing (AAN) experts for the hospitals' reputations for patient care excellence and their ability to attract and retain nurses (McClure, Poulin, Sovie, & Wandelt, 1983), and (2) hospitals designated since 1993 by the American Nurses Credentialing Center's Magnet Hospital Recognition Program.

The original group was selected in 1982 in the midst of a major nursing shortage, after careful scrutiny by AAN nursing administration experts (McClure, Poulin, Sovie, & Wandelt, 1983). AAN fellows nominated 165 acute care hospitals that had reputations for successfully attracting and retaining nurses and for delivering high-quality nursing care. Ultimately, 41 hospitals were selected because they had high rates of nurse satisfaction, low job turnover, and low nurse vacancy rates even when hospitals in close proximity were experiencing nursing high vacancy and turnover rates. These hospitals demonstrated common organizational features, such as

- professional nursing practice models characterized by a high degree of support for nursing care and nurse autonomy
- nurse control over practice
- good communication between nurses and physicians
- a strong, visible, and supportive nursing leadership

Magnet hospital research has provided convincing evidence that into the mid-1990s when the hospital restructuring movement took place, the original magnet hospitals remained institutions where patients received excellent nursing care and where highly qualified professional nurses wished to be employed (Havens & Aiken, 1999; Hinshaw, 2002).

In 1993, the American Nurses Association (ANA), through the American Nurses Credentialing Center (ANCC), established a new magnet hospital designation process, the Magnet Recognition Program. (http://www.ana.org/ancc/magnet.htm#scope). The purpose of the Magnet Recognition Program is to recognize excellence in

- the management, philosophy, and practices of nursing services
- adherence to national standards for high-quality patient care
- leadership of the nurse administrator in supporting professional practice and continued competence of nurses
- understanding and respect for the cultural and ethnic diversity of patients, their significant others, and health care providers

The ANCC magnet recognition process consists of self-nomination, self-appraisal based on the ANCC magnet standards, and a multi-day site visit by trained ANCC appraisers. ANCC magnet hospitals must reapply for magnet status every four years, and they must submit data annually, including ANA Nursing Quality Indicator benchmarking data (NDNQI). According to ANCC, since 1995 all hospitals that have been systematically reevaluated for redesignation by ANCC have achieved magnet status again after four or more years. Those familiar with the self-study associated with the application process report that exploring the nursing structure, the culture, and the interrelationships with other disciplines is a "reforming" experience for the entire organization. Further, they report that self-assessments, benchmarking, defining standards, demonstrating how they meet standards, and empowering "champions" yield positive multilevel, multifunctional organization wide change (Smith, 2002). The Tampa Veterans Administration Hospital reports that "while Magnet recognition is for nursing excellence, it cannot be achieved without hospital-wide involvement." (*VA Call to Action,* p. E2) The report further states, "the application itself is an invaluable learning tool. It forces a detailed self-examination of all aspects of the service from strategic planning to how care is delivered on a daily basis . . . Measuring our practice and performance against the magnet standards has provided a roadmap to improve both our professional performance and care delivery system" (p. E3). As of 2004, over 130 United States hospitals have been recognized as ANCC magnet hospitals, and over 250 applications are in the pipeline (ANCC, personal communication, 2004).

Two decades of research have consistently shown that magnet hospital characteristics are associated with more professional nurse practice environments and better patient and staff outcomes than comparison hospitals (Aiken, Havens, & Sloane, 2000; Havens & Aiken, 1999). Further, the better outcomes cannot be explained by staffing ratios or nurse skill mix alone. Magnet hospitals are characterized by strong organizational and administrative support for the practice of nursing, which enables nurses to use their knowledge to do what they know how to do for patients. This organizational support is critical because nurses are "safety sentinels" (Foley, 2001)—the ongoing hospital surveillance system for the early detection of adverse events, complications, and errors (Aiken, Clarke, & Sloane, 2002). That is, nurses are the providers most likely to identify the early stages of complications or errors, and in some cases they are the providers who are first in line to "rescue" patients (Havens & Aiken, 1999).

Nationally, the magnet hospital model is gaining mainstream policy appeal as a prototype for best practice principles for quality nursing and quality patient care. The model is congruent with recommendations put forward in *Crossing the Quality Chasm* (Institute of Medicine, 2001) to address patient safety through the design of new systems based on professional standards, instituting evidence-based practice, and putting the patient clearly in the picture. It is also congruent with the recommendations in *Keeping Patients Safe: Transforming the Nursing Work Environment of Nurses* (IOM, 2003). In addition, the Nurse Reinvestment Act (PL 107–205) funds nurse education, practice, and retention grants to encourage the implementation of "magnet-like" features in hospitals. In its 2001 report, the VA's National Nursing Workforce Planning Group recommended four domains of intervention to create a more positive work environment for nurses and, thus, increase VA retention of nurses. These domains are addressed in the magnet hospital model. Likewise, the American Hospital Association (2002) and the American Nurses Association (2002) have issued national calls urging the implementation of the organizational features that make magnet hospitals successful. In February 2003, the Joint Commission on Accreditation of Healthcare Organizations established a nursing advisory council to address recommendations from the Joint Commission's white paper *Health Care at the*

Crossroads: Strategies for Addressing the Evolving Nursing Crisis (August, 2002). One recommendation was to implement magnet hospital features.

In summary, while there are several exemplars for the redesign of nursing work, one best practice prototype that is fast gaining international attention is the magnet hospital model. While this model has been associated with nurse recruitment, retention, and quality outcomes for more than 20 years, little is known about how hospitals can successfully implement the model, and even less is known about "how to make it stick." Therefore, the following sections provide compelling stories and key examples of how hospitals have created healthier workplaces by using the magnet principles to redesign nursing work so that nurses and patients can thrive.

EXEMPLAR #1—DEVELOPMENT OF SPECIFIC INITIATIVES TO ACHIEVE MAGNET STATUS IN NEW JERSEY

In the book *The Little Engine That Could,* Watty Piper describes how a little blue train saves the day for the children by being able to get over the hill with the toys. In the story many more powerful trains were asked but they all had excuses and said no. As the little blue train attempted to go over the hill the train was heard saying: "I think I can, I think I can." At the end of the story the train makes it over the hill and said: "I thought I could, I thought I could." This story is reminiscent of what we experienced in our journey. In our first attempt we did not make it, but we did not stop trying until we had success.

Englewood Hospital and Medical Center (EHMC) is a 531-bed community teaching institution. We had had a diploma nursing program since 1896. Because of this arrangement, upon graduation, the majority of nurses went to work at the medical center. Our staff nurses' educational profile was 36% BSN and 64% diploma and associate degree. The average experience of our staff was eight years. The nursing staff had been unionized since the mid-1970s. The first-line managers were long-term employees. Our middle managers were relatively new to the institution. This difference required us to go slowly and understand the belief system.

Our journey began in 1994 with a vision of where we wanted to be, not where we were. We asked ourselves, what do we passionately believe in for nursing at the Medical Center? Passion is key because the hill is steep and a great deal of energy is needed to keep moving forward.

To define our vision we had a two-day retreat. A facilitator was hired to help. We assessed how nursing was being practiced and what was changing in the environment locally, statewide, and nationally. We asked ourselves how nursing was perceived organizationally. We discussed the educational preparation needed for nurses for the future and what the practice model should look like. We began to define goals for the department and identified barriers and obstacles.

We came out of the retreat with three major changes that needed to occur if we were to achieve our vision. These changes were to reposition our school of nursing from a diploma program to a BSN program; to develop a new practice model that focused on education, experience, and competence; and to create our goals around magnet standards.

The leadership team worked together to develop a communication plan for the entire organization. We wrote a white paper on EHMC nursing and formatted it as a brochure so that everyone in the organization would be informed. We identified five-year goals and objectives based on the magnet standards. We developed educational advancement packets and a slide presentation to help communicate the change and provide support. The chief nurse executive took on the task of communicating the change around the clock. The meetings were mandatory. The chief nurse executive had to answer the hard questions and deal with the employees' anger about the new requirement of a BSN for all new hires in the institution. Our audiences for communicating this change were our staff nurses and the union leadership, but we also included the medical leadership, the department managers, administrative staff, and the board of trustees. We needed to ensure that everyone was on board with these changes. If the chief nurse executive is not on board, the project will not succeed. In our case the chief nurse executive was very supportive and committed.

Repositioning the School of Nursing

Institutionally we made a decision to hire only BSN nurses. But how could we educate diploma graduates and not hire them? That would certainly be unethical. It was important that education and practice be aligned. We made a commitment to continue nursing education at the medical center because it was part of our history.

We could not create a BSN program on our own; however, if we partnered with other institutions we could make it cost effective and meet our goals. Our partners are the University of Medicine and

Dentistry of New Jersey, which serves as the parent organization; Ramapo, which provides the science and general education courses, and Englewood Hospital and Medical Center, which teaches all of the nursing courses using our faculty. The partners signed a memorandum of agreement.

We also needed to close our diploma program. So on the 100th-year celebration, we had a massive party, compiled a historical book of the nursing accomplishments, and developed a nursing archival center at the medical center. In 1996 we closed our diploma program and opened our BSN program. A new chapter in nursing education began.

Developing a Professional Practice Model

To create a professional practice model we looked to national organizations and models showing successful outcomes. We utilized the American Association of Colleges of Nursing/American Organization of Nurse Executives 1995 task force recommendations to create our assumptions, with the added assumption that the roles we would develop would be at the bedside. We also used the South Dakota and Colorado models as a framework for differentiated practice. Our practice model includes five components: patient care management, leadership, nursing practice, community outreach, and collaborative practice.

Patient care management is defined by our practice standards, which we formatted based on structure, process, and outcomes. All standards are evidenced based. Compliance with standards is measured by performance improvement activities.

The leadership component defines the expectations of the nursing leadership in facilitating the needs of staff. Each leader in the organization has education and certification expectations. The chief nurse executive expectation is to position nurses as leaders in their field and to be the external liaison for the medical center.

The third component is the practice model itself. This area was the most difficult to implement. First, all new nurses hired from 1995 through 2002 were required to have a BSN. This decision was made based on the recognition that patients were more complex with shorter lengths of stay requiring greater coordination of care. A differentiated practice model was developed, and two RN roles were developed. Staff nurses are required to have a diploma, associate or bachelor's of science in nursing, and they are paid an hourly rate. Staff nurse transfers are based on seniority. The other role is the care manager role. Care managers must have a BSN. They are salaried and considered promotional. Selection for promotion is not by seniority but by qualifications. Both positions are unionized. Additional professional nursing positions in this model include the care coordinator for the unit and the clinical nurse specialist for the specialty.

Community outreach is the fourth component of our model. We identified that practice should go beyond the boundaries of the unit. Nurses make discharge phone calls and participate in health fairs and committees at a state level. The final component is collaborative practice and involves collegiality with other disciplines and team collaboration with support staff.

Creating Goals Around the Magnet Standards

To create the essential elements of magnet status, we utilized the standards as our goals and set objectives that we would meet under each of the standards. For example, under the research goal, we developed a research committee. These goals were shared with the staff.

Developing Outcome Measures/Deliverables

The obvious outcome is receiving magnet status in 2002. However, there are many other outcomes that have been achieved. One is the pride felt by the staff nurses and other disciplines, which is highly evident. In 2002 the nursing research committee received the Sigma Theta Tau Research Dissemination Award, which recognized their work in creating an environment where research is a strong component of professional practice. Recruitment of nurses was also a byproduct. New nurses are looking for practice environments where they can flourish. This reduced our vacancy rate. Retention continues to be a strong attribute of our organization. Currently 66% of our staff nurses and care managers who have a BSN are working at the bedside. This had a positive impact on the environment, especially on patient care, although this has not been quantitatively measured. The final lesson is that you never can go back to where you were. The staff and managers are seeking to build and move practice, education, and research forward.

We asked our staff what made EHMC a place they wanted to practice. They said things like "I feel connected immediately," "I don't feel like a number," "I can be a nurse," "My voice is heard," and "Leadership is involved with staff nurses." They also identified advantages such as the opportunities for growth, flexible scheduling, benefits, working with experienced and competent staff, the professional environment, management accessibility, the internship program, being part of decision making, and a family environment.

Obstacles Encountered, Lessons Learned

Our first attempt failed. We had an unfair labor practice by our nursing union that took too long to resolve. Several people wrote our application, and that method was not successful. One person needs to edit and a small team needs to write the application. Also there will always be those who believe they are not ready. Go with the majority of staff who are positive. Seven years is a long journey, but it was well worth the trip. The journey, however, is not over. It continues as we move to the next level of practice. We thought we could. We thought we could.

EXEMPLAR #2—REDESIGN OF NURSING WORK AT A RURAL HOSPITAL IN SOUTH DAKOTA

The honest way to describe the medical/surgical care model at Prairie Lakes Healthcare System before changes were made was as the Fragmented Total Patient Care. In addition, the detail of every job was codified to the extent that the ability to initiate change, think critically, and improve job satisfaction was impaired.

Inpatient care delivery systems include many subsystems: the admission system, the staffing system, the documentation system, the discharge system, the care team roles and responsibilities system, the critical-thinking system, and the human cultural system. The fragmented total patient care model, caused problems with all of these subsystems. For Prairie Lakes, the bedside care delivery model remained essentially unchanged for 20 years even though the health care environment had changed dramatically during this time: Length of stay was down, patient days were up, hospital margins were compromised, and the workforce was unhappy and aging. Work intensity in the acute care hospital continued to rise and was a major source of frustration for the workforce.

This exemplar of redesigning nursing work illustrates how one organization approached system problems and transitioned to a contemporary, team, patient-care model. The transition began four years ago, focusing on fundamentals such as leadership, staffing and scheduling, documentation systems, and work process. Today, Prairie Lakes has a new model responsive to the care delivery challenges of the present environment.

Portrait of a Small Community Hospital

Prairie Lakes Healthcare System is a small, independent, nonprofit community hospital located in Watertown, South Dakota (population 20,000). Even though licensed for only 81 beds, it is distinctly different from the prototype rural hospital known as the critical access hospital. It has an 8-bed critical care unit, 52 operational medical/surgical beds, and an obstetrics service with 500 births per year. The hospital operates a full-service cancer center that includes radiation therapy and four dialysis units with rural satellites. The system includes a 55-bed long-term care facility and a home health agency. The closest tertiary-care center is 100 miles away. Prairie Lakes is not a rural hospital but a rural regional medical center that provides all but the most tertiary services.

Like most small, independent hospitals left in America, the hospital is financially sound, reporting a net income of $5 million on revenue of $65 million for 2003. The medical staff include 50 active staff physicians representing a number of medical specialties. Four years ago, there were serious problems with staffing and workforce satisfaction on the medical/surgical unit. The unit's turnover rate was 65%. The registered nurse vacancy rate was 29%. The organization did not use agency staff or float staff from other internal nursing departments, and therefore vacancies had to be covered by an already stressed and undersized workforce. Staff were frequently mandated to work additional hours and shifts. About two-thirds of the nursing staff had less than 3 years of experience. It was not uncommon to see a nurse leave the job—and the organization—within one year of initial employment.

An employee opinion survey completed in the summer 2000 showed that, on the medical/surgical unit, staff's overall satisfaction was 50% lower than that of the overall hospital staff. Complaints about the work environment focused on leadership and work activities that were considered complex, wasteful, or demoralizing. "That's just the way it is on a medical/surgical unit," said an employee. "It's an entry-level unit. No one wants to work there. The work is so hard. You just put in your time until you can transfer to an easy unit like obstetrics (OB) or coronary care unit (CCU)."

In addition, there were problems with the care delivery model, and bedside staff wanted change. A charge nurse without a patient assignment was responsible for rounding with physicians, processing physician orders, reviewing lab work, and contacting physicians to report changes in patient condition. The charge nurse made patient assignments to licensed nursing staff responsible for the start-to-finish direct patient-care needs of each assigned patient. The bedside nurse had minimal accountability for patient outcomes, clinical decision making, managing care, or directing the care activities of other nursing staff and health professionals. Registered nurse case managers, who did not have a direct role in providing patient care, were responsible for coordinating activities related to discharge, such as arranging long-term care placement. Other members of the patient-care team were seldom involved in discharge planning. Finally, the unit was not operating cost effectively. With high turnover and ineffective staffing, labor costs were high. Resources were being consumed to support a dysfunctional staffing system rather than addressing waste, inefficiency, and cost of services.

Prior to making changes in the bedside care delivery model, issues in the work environment related to leadership and staffing were addressed. In addition, it was important to leverage new information technology adopted in June 2002 and streamline documentation.

Leadership Reorganization: Decreasing Span of Control

The nurse manager of the troubled medical/surgical unit was responsible not only for the direction of the medical/surgical unit but also the OB unit. An assistant manager was assigned to each unit to support the nurse manager. A new nurse executive hired in June 2000 decided the medical/surgical unit required a dedicated, visible nurse manager who could focus on the issues of the department. To avoid adding full-time staff, the assistant managers were transferred back to open staff nurse positions, and the incumbent medical/surgical director was reassigned to exclusive nurse manager duties for the OB unit. Because the OB unit was small (14 full-time equivalents), part of her time was allocated to direct patient-care activities. A new medical/surgical manager with an employee-centered style of leadership was hired. Two years after the new leader was hired, a repeat employee opinion survey showed a 50% improvement in the overall job satisfaction score on the medical/surgical unit.

Staffing System Revision: Central Control and Cross-Training

A project team with representatives from each nursing unit was established in fall 2000 to revise the nursing staffing system in order to meet the following objectives: meet patient needs as demands increase or decrease, and align unit staffing plans with the hospital staffing system. The team focused on patient census staffing, patient classification and workload systems, and scheduling policies and practices. The recommendations to alleviate staffing problems included floating, a practice that had not been required and was viewed negatively by nurses in specialty units. The team believed that floating was the most effective way to alleviate the crisis on the medical/surgical unit. In addition, the team recommended the elimination of mandatory overtime, centralization and standardization of daily staffing, and development of float competencies. Within a year, turnover on the medical/surgical unit was down 25% and staff stated that they were experiencing less stress related to working extra shifts. Now staffing needs were collectively met by nurses from all inpatient units rather than relying solely on the resources of the medical/surgical unit. Staffing flexibility was a major factor contributing to improved productivity. The medical/surgical unit hours per patient day went from a high of 11.5 to 8.2 in 2004.

Documentation Revision:
Transition to an Efficient Electronic Health Record

During the process of selecting a new information system to be implemented in June 2002, the organization was surprised to learn that electronic documentation did not always save time. Studies indicate 30 minutes of documentation are required for every hour of patient care on a medical/surgical unit, and Prairie Lakes wanted to address this major source of inefficiency. The organization challenged the assumption that documentation time would not be reduced by fundamentally redesigning the existing documentation system. The health record was redefined, and wasteful documentation activities were eliminated. Transition to an electronic health record continues and is now integrated with the initiative to change the care delivery model.

Rethinking Care Delivery

In January 2003, the hospital initiated a project team called Work Matters to redesign the care delivery model on the medical/surgical unit. The project was regarded as a workforce development project to emphasize issues that were critical for staff satisfaction and retention.

The aim of the project was to improve the work environment of the medical/surgical unit by implementing a new care delivery model that decreased work intensity and improved staff satisfaction, driven by the following broad goals:

• Generate new ideas that could be pilot tested for use in a redesigned care delivery model.
• Determine the most appropriate configuration, roles, and competencies of the patient care team.
• Simplify and standardize tasks to eliminate waste.
• Redesign patient flow and care coordination during the hospital stay.

Specific metrics and targets were developed to measure the following objectives:

• Reduce waste in patient care processes.
• Increase the amount of time nurses spend in direct patient care activities.
• Improve staff satisfaction.
• Reduce staff turnover.
• Maintain nurse-patient ratios comparable to proposed ratios (industry).
• Reduce day-shift overtime hours (an indicator of work intensity).
• Meet established productivity standards.

The project team also developed metrics to better understand the current environment. For example, an admission, discharge, and transfer rate (ADT index) was measured to provide a better understanding of the work intensity related to patient turnover.

Methodologically, the project team was educated about workforce issues, care delivery models, and best practices. The organization joined an Institute for Healthcare Improvement (IHI) breakthrough collaborative, Achieving Workforce Excellence, to develop changes in the management process and gain best practice knowledge on creating positive work environments. Using the IHI model of rapid-cycle change and pilot testing, the team developed and implemented a number of changes in the care delivery model and work environment. In addition, the team was influenced by lean engineering principles from the Toyota production system because of the emphasis on designing processes to eliminate waste. The testing model is summarized in Figure 5.1.

Pilot testing was accomplished by designating a 10-bed section of the 52 licensed medical/surgical beds as the test site. The pilot was

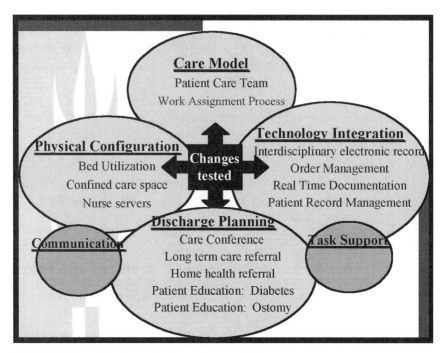

FIGURE 5.1   Testing of a new care model.

initiated in April 2003 with a reconfigured patient care team. The results of the pilot project were disseminated to the entire medical/surgical department in July 2003. Through the pilot and full implementation phase, the team tested over 50 changes and refined the model through a series of Plan-Do-Study-Act (PDSA) cycles (see examples in Figures 5.2 and 5.3).

A team nursing concept was implemented with an RN care manager and two other providers to care for a cohort ranging from 10 to 12 patients. The care manager functioned as both a provider and a manager of care, assuming overall responsibilities for the performance of the bedside nursing team, clinical outcomes of patients, coordination of patient care processes, and supervision of patient care processes. Essential principles of the team model were adapted from a Health Care Advisory Board model and included the following: (1) Every patient deserves to be cared for by an experienced RN. (2) Every patient assigned to the team belongs to each team member. (3) Team members function within their defined roles, scope of practice, and competencies.

The team composition and work process changed depending on daily staffing and patient census. For example, the care manager

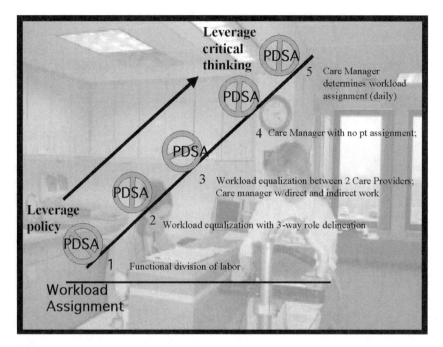

FIGURE 5.2 Testing changes to the work assignment process—patient care team.

might lead a team consisting of two other experienced licensed nurses and have minimal direct supervision responsibilities. On the other hand, the team might include a new graduate nurse and a float nurse uncomfortable with a patient assignment. In this case, the care manager would determine the best approach such as delegation of patient care tasks to the float nurse and mentoring of the new graduate.

As the testing of the team and leadership roles progressed, it became clear that the care manager needed more critical-thinking and problem-solving skills than were needed with the prescriptive policies of the past in order to guide decisions about patient assignments and managing patient care. Care managers also assumed responsibility for managing the interdisciplinary discharge plan and were expected to conduct a daily interdisciplinary team conference for their patient cohort. Staff were initially uncomfortable with the new degree of accountability, and developing the required skill set continues to be challenging because these roles are typically assumed by advanced practice nurses in larger health care organizations.

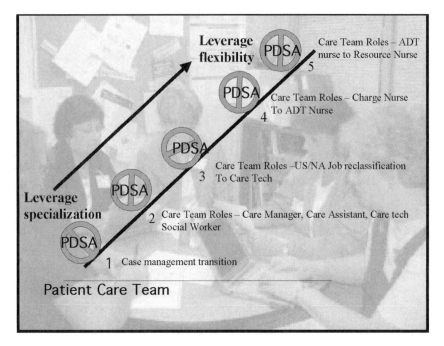

FIGURE 5.3   Testing changes to the team model.

Innovations with Impact

Streamlined Documentation

Through further development of the electronic health record and redesign of documentation practices, nursing time spent in managing documentation was reduced by 50%. Documentation revision projects included eliminating the traditional care plan, revising discharge and transfer documentation, and revising consent documentation.

Getting Nurses Back to the Patient

Nursing positions on the medical/surgical unit that were not related to direct patient care were eliminated (e.g., discharge planners and charge nurses without patient assignments). By redirecting staff resources, the unit was able to maintain average nurse to patient ratios of 1:4 on the day shift without adding to overall labor cost. In addition, staff with direct care responsibilities were required to participate in discharge planning, which improved the overall effectiveness of the process.

Skills Realignment

Job expectations for registered nurses have been elevated to optimize role function. The role includes leading an interdisciplinary team, and more actively delegating and supervising the work of others. The team approach to care is efficient, but strong team leadership is essential to success. The roles of other nursing team members have also been developed. Nursing assistants and licensed practical nurses are better utilized with more effective delegation and skills training. A resource nurse position has also been created (without adding full-time staff) by eliminating the traditional charge nurse role. The resource nurse provides bed control, initiates patient admissions, and provides support for advanced nursing procedures under the direction of the RN team leaders. This has reduced the bedside nursing team's work intensity associated with admission activity.

Real-Time Daily Care Conferences

The entire discharge planning process was redesigned with the introduction of the daily care conference. Every morning, team members from nursing, social work, home health, physical therapy, dietary, and pastoral care conduct a brief review of each patient's discharge plan. On average, the discussion is limited to one minute per patient, and team members identify any needs for more extended discussions. The conference information is immediately entered into the patient's electronic record, which improves access to critical information for all providers.

Outsourced Order Management

Overall, the medical/surgical unit functions with the same number of unit secretary full-time equivalents, but redesign has created more nursing wings secondary to team configurations. In addition, all unit secretaries have been crossed-trained to participate in patient-care activities. Due to these factors, the capacity for processing patient orders is occasionally challenged. Using information technology, the organization has designed a system for orders to be processed by unit secretaries in other units with lower workloads.

Summary and Lessons Learned

Through a series of innovations that evolved through testing based on principles of rapid-cycle change and lean engineering, an entire care delivery model that had been in place for years was redesigned in less than one year. Several lessons learned are of note:

- The problems on the medical/surgical unit were accepted as the status quo until there was a crisis that led to recognition of the problems. Unfortunately, this may be happening in many American hospitals. *Lesson:* Life on the medical/surgical unit can be improved.
- Change of this magnitude may result in unpopular decisions that are met with the response "People will quit if we do that!" *Lesson:* There are fewer quitters than you think.
- Innovation means radical redesign of a process. We are not there yet in the transformation of patient-care delivery models. *Lesson:* We are trapped in so many traditions that often we cannot see our opportunities.
- Work-intensity problems cannot be fixed by simply adding more staff. Also, there are not enough nurses, and we all have a role in being good stewards of our scarce and costly resources. *Lesson:* We have to change the way we work.
- Registered nurses in traditional bedside staff nurse roles are capable of effectively leading the interdisciplinary team. *Lesson:* We need to commit to leadership at the bedside and develop the professional role of the hospital staff RN.
- Acute-care nursing is never static, and the situation the care team has to deal with is different every day. *Lesson:* It is more essential to think critically than to complete tasks to meet the challenges in this environment.
- Teamwork dynamics affect how well challenges are met. *Lesson:* In addition to work redesign, training, education, development, and good leadership, attitude counts.

The new model is responsive to changes that have occurred over the past two decades in American hospitals. It is affordable, work intensity has decreased, and workforce satisfaction has improved. For Prairie Lakes, the work is continuing, and future initiatives are planned to develop the bedside nursing leader and explore the "brave new world" of acuity adaptable beds.

EXEMPLAR #3—IMPLEMENTATION OF RESEARCH ON WORKPLACE ISSUES IN GREATER KANSAS CITY

This exemplar is about creating and sustaining a research program on the work environment of nurses. The research program was built on the contributions of Linda Aiken, Peter Buerhaus, and others who have championed the scientific approach for this area. They have taken the emotion out of an emotionally charged issue. And they have challenged all of us, whether in service or the academic environment, to collaborate the creation of meaningful and actionable research projects yielding data that will scientifically support changing the face of health care for the betterment of nurses and the patients they serve.

Specifically, this exemplar analyzes completed studies that used a deductive approach in health care environmental research. Each study builds on the preceding work to refine the questions asked and to generate new knowledge. First, the results of a single-hospital study on occupational stress and coping for inpatient nurses is followed by the results of a multicenter duplication. The second study uses a new, valid and reliable instrument to assess nurses' perception of workload through a series of support factors within an organization and their intent to stay at the institution. Again, research was conducted in a single institution followed by a multisite study. Following these results will be a synthesis of new knowledge gained, implications of the research, and a charge to leaders for future directions.

The Magnet Recognition Program and the components of magnet organizations provided the underpinnings and rationale for this work. Nurses as well as patients in these settings are more satisfied and have better outcomes. A national strategy for our health care system is firmly established financial incentives that reward institutions seeking this designation. Institutions lacking the infrastructure to achieve all the characteristics of magnet status should be assisted, through partnerships with participating hospitals, to achieve this worthy goal.

In addition, formal programs like the Robert Wood Johnson Greater Kansas City Colleagues in Caring (CIC) project serve as a venue for dialogue among leaders in the academic and service organizations for nursing. They also serve as the ideal platform for recruitment of study participants for research projects from service organizations (i.e., inpatient nurses) and a sound environment for regional dissemination of these findings. These collaborations continue to thrive well after the formal structure has ended.

Final thoughts will center on the unprecedented need for those in service and academic environments to build mutually beneficial, symbiotic programs of research that center around the nursing work environment. In her book, *Becoming Influential: A Guide for Nurses,* Eleanor Sullivan (2003) outlines strategies for nurses using the principle of quid pro quo—what each can do for one another.

Although Sullivan extends the concept beyond service-academic potential, the principle is as relevant in this domain as in other potential alliances. The service-academic partnership is one that can leverage the power of academic science and the reality of the service setting to produce outstanding possibilities to influence the greater good and impact policy. That greater good is improving the professional lives of nurses and the care of patients. For many in both sectors, however, these collaborations remain illusive. It is critical for the survival of nursing that these alliances be forged to create information so undeniably compelling that not only will individual organizations institute change, but national policy makers will become engaged in this dialogue to create minimum standards of practice for those who care for our nation's people.

Describing Occupational Stress, Strain, and Coping for Inpatient Nurses

Single-Hospital Study

The Santos and Cox (2000) study marked the first published results from a research study that found baby-boomer nurses (those born between 1946 and 1964) had more stress and less effective coping than did other age cohorts. Prior to this work there was only anecdotal information and marketing literature highlighting baby boomers and their response in interacting with other cohorts, most specifically generation Xers. In addition, it was the first documented study using only nurses that found these significant differences.

To assess the current status of occupational adjustment, the Occupational Stress Inventory (OSI) was administered to 413 nurses from 16 nursing units at a large pediatric hospital in the Midwest after human subjects approval (Osipow & Spokane, 1981). Data were collected at mandatory unit meetings; however, participation in the study was optional.

The study included 68% of the hospital's total nursing workforce, of whom 70% were full-time employees. The OSI, a 140-item five-point Likert scale instrument, addresses occupational stress, strain, and coping with 15 scales subsumed within the whole. All scales have alpha coefficients ranging from 0.71 to 0.94 and therefore are considered a good indicator of the concepts under investigation (Polit & Hungler, 1997). Analysis of variance or t-tests were used, and the appropriate post hoc tests employed when indicated. Significance levels for all analyses were set at $p = .05$.

Of the 413 nurses in the sample, 4.1% were of the mature genera-tion (born 1909–1945), 43% were baby boomers (born 1946–1964), and 41% were Xers (born 1965–1981). The aggregate results of the OSI revealed all stress, strain, and coping scales within normal ranges compared with the normative data. However, the investigators believed there was opportunity for improvement. The most prob-lematic scales within the stress and strain inventory for this sample appear in Table 5.1, in descending order.

Baby boomers had significantly higher mean scores on stress scales of role overload and role boundary. Matures had the highest mean scores for role insufficiency and gen Xers had the highest mean scores on physical environment. In strain subscales, baby boomers had higher mean scores for vocational strain and interper-sonal strain. Baby-boomer nurses had lower mean scores for the subscales of self-care and social support, whereas the mature nurses had the highest mean scores on the same subscales.

Analysis of these data provided the framework for the semi-structured interview questions. Inquiries centered on further expla-nation of the findings of the survey. Ten focus groups were held over a two-month period at various shifts and on the weekend. Focus groups were conducted using semistructured interviews to clarify the findings of the OSI. Ten focus groups were held over a two-month period with a total sample of 44 registered nurses in attendance.

Nurses who participated in the survey were asked to attend the focus group of their choice and to identify specific examples of how a defined subscale plays out on their unit. These groups were held until saturation with themes occurred. Nurses were exceptionally forth-coming.

Three system themes were identified: workplace design, per-sonnel needs, and communication (inter- and intradepartmental).

Given the significant differences found with the survey linked to age cohorts, it was important to explore generational themes. It was evident during the focus groups that baby boomers' distress with younger workers was palpable. The three themes identified in the focus groups were orientation toward work (baby boomers did not believe younger nurses were sufficiently committed to the profes-sion, the unit, or the patients; turnover (baby boomers perceived a "revolving door" of new nurses and disliked training new nurses only to have them leave for "greener pastures" after a short while); and workplace behavior (baby boomers felt that younger nurses were arrogant and self-absorbed and not as "team focused" as they were). By striking contrast, gen X nurses did not express intense negative beliefs about either baby boomer or mature nurses.

TABLE 5.1 Significant Differences Between Generations: Stress, Strain, and Coping Scales (OSI)

Scale	Mean (SD)	T-Score	Normal T-score range	Significance
Stress scales (Higher scores are more negative.)				
Role overload				
• Generation Xers	24.27 (5.20)	49	40–59	.018
• Baby boomers	25.75 (6.21)	50		
• Matures	22.88 (4.80)	46		
Role insufficiency				
• Generation Xers	18.96 (5.37)	43	40–59	.000
• Baby boomers	21.49 (6.20)	45		
• Matures	21.82 (3.41)	46		
Physical environment				
• Generation Xers	23.26 (4.81)	57	40–59	.040
• Baby boomers	22.79 (7.03)	57		
• Matures	18.82 (6.80)	52		
Role boundary				
• Generation Xers	20.55 (5.36)	49	40–59	.041
• Baby boomers	21.64 (6.20)	51		
• Matures	18.47 (5.36)	50		

TABLE 5.1 *(Continued)*

Scale	Mean (SD)	T-Score	Normal T-score range	Significance
Strain scales (Higher scores are more negative.)				
Vocational strain				
• Generation Xers	15.98 (4.01)	45	40–59	.017
• Baby boomers	17.34 (4.81)	47		
• Matures	17.23 (5.30)	47		
Interpersonal strain				
• Generation Xers	19.48 (5.37)	45	40–59	.020
• Baby boomers	20.69 (5.98)	48		
• Matures	17.35 (4.03)	42		
Coping scales (*Lower* scores are more negative.)				
Self-care				
• Generation Xers	25.81 (5.80)	47	40–59	.010
• Baby boomers	24.98 (6.52)	46		
• Matures	29.70 (7.05)	53		
Social support				
• Generation Xers	42.03 (6.52)	52	40–59	.001
• Baby boomers	39.48 (7.85)	48		
• Matures	43.58 (6.12)	54		

However, they did at times feel the negativity from baby boomer's toward them in subtle and not-so-subtle ways. Matures nurses believed they had "been there, done that" and were witnessing situations they had encountered throughout their careers.

Interventions. In an effort to create interventions for nurses that addressed these specific problems, a two-phase approach was used. In phase two, each of three interventions addressed the needs identified in both the survey and focus group results. Key informant nurses were consulted in creating the interventions with the management team. Interventions included the following: (1) An internal transport team was created so that nurses need not abandon their colleagues and patients to accompany a patient for procedures. (2) The use of technology (phones and pagers) was increased where feasible. Phones and pagers allowed nurses to be reached and to reach others, reducing the feeling of poor communication, especially in units where the architecture was not conducive for good communication (nursing pods within the unit as a whole). Unit secretaries were also provided with better guidelines for phone triage of incoming calls that constantly interrupted them given care. (3) Staffing was increased with a voluntary on-call pool for intermittent peak needs, especially admissions and discharges.

The phase two intervention was a three-part educational series covering managed care and its impact on health care, personal stress and coping assessments and relevant interventions, and generational values clarification over a one-year period provided to nursing units.

Multisite Duplication

A multisite duplication followed general discussions of the preceding findings through joint meetings between service and academic leaders in the Greater Kansas City Colleagues in Caring initiative in which the authors of this chapter were integrally involved. The work was continued through a Robert Wood Johnson Executive Nurse Fellowship as a large-scale effort to help other area nurse executives assess their work environment in order to make substantial improvements. A call for participation yielded several institutions wishing to participate in a multisite duplication of the initial study using the same methodology that is, the OSI followed by focus groups (Santos, Carroll, et al., 2003).

The duplication study was carried out at three diverse institutions in the Midwest—one rural, one urban, and one suburban site—and a final participant number of 694 inpatient nurses. Data analysis included the initial site in the aforementioned study. Of the 694 participants, there were 55 mature nurses (8%), 368 baby-boomer nurses (53%), and 246 generation X nurses (35%).

Baby-boomer nurses had significantly higher (more negative) stress scores than their colleagues in the two other age cohorts of matures and generation Xers. Significant results included role overload (p = .043), role boundary (p = .023), role ambiguity (p = .030); role insufficiency (p = .001); and physical environment (p = .000). The definitions of the findings are as follows: Baby boomers again had significantly more interpersonal strain than other cohorts (p = .015). On two of the three coping subscales, baby boomer respondents had significantly worse scores (poorer coping) than participants in the other age cohorts. These subscales were self-care (p = .002) and social support (p = 004).

After the analysis was performed on the OSI-R, focus groups were conducted to clarify the findings. The results indicated that problems associated with key stressors in the workplace could be grouped into three themes: unit "speed up" (admissions, discharges, and transfers) and the use of staffing calculations that did not factor in these activities, the pressure to provide customer service and quality care, and staff shortages. After the findings were reported back to each facility, the authors worked with the senior nurse executive, formally or informally, to create meaningful interventions for their hospitals.

Both studies offered undeniable congruence about the chaotic work environment and generational differences, raising the level of awareness about this problem to new heights in the region. Subsequent dialogue through the CIC program provided the ideal venue for best practices and interventions to be discussed.

Measuring Nurses' Support, Workload, and Intent to Stay

As previously indicated, the program of research used deductive logic in the approach to fully describe the work environment for nurses. The aforementioned studies provided a framework for the general understanding of the inpatient nurse's work setting, particularly in stress, strain, and coping. This study refined these stress concepts more fully by gaining understanding of the support structures and nurses' perceptions of workload in an organization that account for nurses wanting to stay in a particular job. The instrument used was created especially for this refined approach in ascertaining specific support factors that most influence this intent to stay and was built on the work of Aiken and Patrician (2000) Advisory Board documents about support for frontline workers.

First, the Individual Workload Perception Scale (IWPS) is explained—particularly, its validity and reliability. Second, the results of two studies using the scale are presented.

Workload as a concept is extremely complex and is inherently based on the nurse's perception of his or her environment and personal skills. Attempts to measure workload have primarily focused on objective measures such as hours per patient day or acuity based on concrete nursing tasks. Workload, as measured with surrogates such as hours per patient day or acuity, however, is simply not sufficient to capture the essence of the comoplex inpatient environment in today's inpatient setting. Those objective measures only provide part of the equation of workload. Workload also involves organizational support factors that do or do not support the staff nurse's practice. Therefore it is critical to capture these complementary factors simultaneously with workload in order to provide a more comprehensive picture and provide actionable data for those charged with managing health care resources. These complementary factors pertinent to the staff nurse's perception of workload are unit, peer, organizational, and manager support.

Finally, any such instrument sensitive enough to capture the complex factors of workload and support factors objectively must be linked to yet another concept: intent to stay. Understanding the relationship between these factors and the intent to stay in the inpatient health care environment can make the difference about where scarce resources are spent to improve the environmental for nurses.

The Individual Workload Perception Scale was created with these complex factors in mind. The theoretical model for the IWPS is based on the notion that workload perception is made up of five concepts: manager support (MS), peer support (PS), unit support (US), nursing satisfaction (NS), and intent to stay (ITS). The theoretical underpinnings of the support factors (MS, PS, and US) translate into satisfaction or dissatisfaction with the inpatient workplace. Intent to stay is a reaction to this satisfaction or dissatisfaction. The five concepts are as follows:

- Manager support is the extent to which supervisors or managers provide help and serve as a resource in the work group. This support can take many forms. A nurse manager who is clinically competent and available may rarely need to provide direct nursing care as long as nurses believe this support exists. A nurse manager who is empathetic about workload issues and appears to work hard at filling open positions will also positively influence workload perception.

- Peer support is the extent to which there is cohesion in the work group. It is the extent to which teamwork exists.
- Unit support includes the necessary tools to do the job at hand, patient care. It also includes support and assistance with important but not necessarily clinical tasks such as secretarial support.
- Intent to stay reflects the nurse's cognitive intent to stay with an organization, in particular, the present position.
- Nursing satisfaction is an aggregate measure of the other variables.

An instrument such as the IWPS, a 46-item, Likert-scale survey instrument is comprehensive with sound psychometric properties. It takes less than 15 minutes to administer and can provide actionable information for managers and health care executives to use in improving the environment for our direct care providers. Initial testing of the instrument has found it to have twice the predictive capabilities of typical scales used currently to measure intent to leave, and it is geared specifically for inpatient nurses.

The pilot study was conducted with a sample of inpatient registered nurses at a large urban hospital (187 beds) in the Midwest (N = 687) using the IWPS. AMOS, a structural equation modeling software program, was used to analyze the data.

Nurses with more manager, peer, and unit support and who perceived they had reasonable workloads were more likely to have scores reflecting the intent to stay. In addition, in multiple linear regression models, combined manager, peer, unit, and workload accounted for 45% of the total variance for intent to stay. This percentage is twice the usual success of similar types of instruments in defining the end point variable. In other words, the user can be more than reasonably sure of the information gleaned from the IWPS to predict the intent to stay.

A larger scale study was conducted at the statewide level in Missouri. Names and addresses of registered nurses were purchased from the state board of nursing. After the names were stratified by Zip code and mailed, 769 nurses completed the survey, and 691 indicated they were working in the nursing field. Data from the 691 working nurses were analyzed.

Mature nurse composed 9%, baby boomers; 63%; generation Xers, 27%; and a new generation, generation Y (born after 1980), was 1% of the sample. Manager and peer support and workload are directly influential for intent to stay; whereas manager, peer, and unit support are indirectly influential on intent to stay. All data were analyzed using AMOS. Nursing satisfaction was most influenced by the shift on which nurses worked. Day-shift nurses were more satisfied that nurses on night shift or alternative shifts. In addition, nurses who worked in specialty areas were more satisfied than those who worked on general units.

SYNTHESIS OF RESEARCH

These studies have contributed significantly to our knowledge about nurses currently working in today's inpatient environment. Using a general to specific approach, it has been determined that nurses' stress is increased in baby boomer-nurses, the largest group of nurses working today. In addition, they generally cope less effectively than other age groups who work with them. Intergenerational conflict adds strain to an already stressful workplace. The overwhelming burden placed on baby-boomer nurses as the seasoned professionals at the bedside provides an increased specter of dissonance as they try to reconcile how things were with how they are now.

We know also that nurses need tangible support in the workplace. Organizational factors such as manager, unit, and peer support create the right combination for nurses to function professionally. These support factors contribute significantly to whether nurses want to stay or leave an organization. The use of a diagnostic tool can provide actionable data for nurse executives to create interventions targeted on the right sector of the workplace.

THE CASE FOR COLLABORATION

Perhaps the greatest lesson we can learn from this body of work and the landmark body of work of Linda Aiken is that regardless of what outside consultants may tell us about the health care workplace, the best and most reliable source for this critical information is the nurses themselves. Creating change without their input would be similar to building a boat in order to sail the desert.

The studies presented here could not have been completed without the generous participation of the inpatient nurses and administrators from all of the organizations studied. The program of research continues to grow and has generated new knowledge and helped change regional competitors into champions for nurses at the bedside. Working together, we built a minimum standard of practice throughout the region that is reflected in how decisions are made. This alliance is not unusual and can be replicated in other regions. It takes an agreement about the common ground on which to base decisions about how information will be used and shared. If collaborators can institute these decisions, there is no limit to where such research can take us.

6

Innovations in Nursing Education

Brenda Cleary, Susan A. Boyer,
Claudia Johnston, and Renatta S. Loquist

INTRODUCTION

Discussions of nursing workforce issues generally focus on the numbers of nurses needed to meet health care needs. However, optimal nursing resources are only realized when the nursing workforce is both adequate in numbers and preparation for delivering nursing services in an increasingly complex health care environment. Therefore, a visionary approach to nursing education is critical to assuring the nursing workforce of the future.

EXEMPLAR #1—THE NORTH CAROLINA EXPERIENCE

Recent groundbreaking research by Aiken, Clarke, Cheung, Sloane, and Silber (2003) shows an inverse relationship between the educational levels of nurses and patient mortality and failure to rescue. The educational preparation of the nursing workforce continues to be a conundrum for the nursing profession. Sometimes, it is necessary to look for the second or even the third or fourth right answers.

As part of its mission to ensure that North Carolina has the nursing resources to meet the health care needs of its citizens, the North Carolina Center for Nursing sponsored a think tank from 2000 to 2002 for creating a shared vision for nursing's preferred future in North Carolina. Participants in think tank activities included nursing leaders from nursing education at all levels, the multiple sectors of the health care industry, professional associations, the North Carolina Area Health Education Center Program, the North Carolina Board of Nursing, and the North Carolina Center for Nursing.

The North Carolina Nurse FutureThink was guided by Vision 2020 and developed by a coalition of national nursing organizations. The challenge was to develop a comprehensive plan for nursing practice, education, and credentialing that (1) distinguishes the specific sets of competencies that will be needed for the profession to meet its social mandate to improve health and provide care and (2) ensures that nursing is developed as a career that will attract a sufficient supply of new entrants necessary to meet the needs of society.

Collective Vision of Nursing in the 21st Century

Nursing develops and utilizes a strong knowledge base and the flexibility to apply knowledge in a wide variety of care settings along an integrated continuum of care from wellness and prevention to episodic illness and, in some cases, through chronicity. Nurses are committed to all aspects of health care planning and delivery wherever members of society experience health- and illness-related events. Nursing is driven by critical thinking and problem solving to identify, measure, and achieve the best possible outcome for the patient.

The discipline must clearly and visibly demonstrate a unique expertise and body of knowledge, participate actively in policy making, perform an essential public good, achieve control and autonomy, ensure commitment to the profession and a professional culture, and agree on a code of ethics. Nursing must incorporate (1) professional and ethical principles that demonstrate an understanding of fiscal accountability and responsibility that lead to cost-effective care delivery in the setting most appropriate to meet the patient's needs and (2) the ability to work collaboratively within an interdisciplinary framework and foster team processes without territorial bias in order to best serve the patient.

Nursing requires strong skills in assessment, definitive nursing diagnosis, individualized care planning, identification and delivery of appropriate patient-specific interventions, patient and family education, and communication with individuals, patients, and populations. Nursing manages health care with the consumer and partners with the individual in the development of a wellness plan. Nursing requires mastery of information systems and biomedical technology. Nursing also requires the ability to assimilate and process data from multiple sources to (1) plan and coordinate a program of nursing care that effectively addresses individual and family needs from a holistic perspective and (2) delegate to other care providers appropriately. Recommended core competencies for nursing education include

- ethics (includes advocacy)
- cultural competence
- decision making, application, and synthesis (includes assessment skills)
- research and evidence-based practice (monitoring, treatment, and educational interventions)
- health care delivery/economics
- leadership and management (delegation and supervision)
- health policy
- teaching/learning
- informatics
- communication (oral and written)
- caring/interpersonal skills
- psychomotor skills
- regulatory competence, including legal issues, safety, and risk management
- professional socialization (includes history of nursing)

The model for nursing education reform that evolved from FutureThink was a competency-based model in which, beginning with the associate's degree, each level of nursing education built on the previous by increasing the degree of autonomy and the degree of complexity/specificity of each competency. The competency-based model allowed for a differentiation of licensure, roles, and compensation. However, as the early model was released, the political fallout from multiple stakeholders was enormous.

Virtually all of the fallout related to FutureThink centered on levels I and II (AD, BSN) with little attention to innovation proposed at the graduate level. The National Advisory Council on Nursing Education and Practice recommended to the Division of Nursing that we work to change the proportion of the registered nursing workforce from 60% with less than a baccalaureate degree to 60% with at least a BSN degree. To ensure a more highly educated workforce, perhaps we need to consider a different and in some ways bolder challenge: that by 2020, 60% of our national registered nursing workforce be RNs with some sort of undergraduate preparation (AD, BSN) and that 40% be at least master's prepared.

Perhaps we need to rejuvenate the clinical nurse specialist (CNS) role, as it was originally conceptualized, i.e., the expert nurse at the bedside or the patient's side. These nurses would be charged with working with a team of staff nurses in providing continuity of nursing care that is safer and more satisfying for patients and their families. These nurses would also be charged with being the retention officers of the future and with facilitating the transition of new graduates to the workplace. No new means of licensing/credentialing would be required beyond the existing legal recognition of the CNS, unlike, but otherwise similar to, the clinical nurse leader role being proposed by the American Association of Colleges of Nursing.

However, reclaiming and increasing the prevalence of the role will require strengthening the evidence base regarding improved patient outcomes and cost effectiveness. And, of course, the 40% of the RN workforce with graduate preparation would also include faculty, administrators, researchers, policy experts, informatics experts, and other types of advanced practice nurses.

A group of nurse executives, nurse educators, advanced practice nurses, and students was recently convened with funding from the Robert Wood Johnson Executive Nurse Fellow program. Assisted by a doctoral student research assistant and representatives of a local college interested in piloting a new model, Brenda Cleary led the group to develop the following template for an entry-level master's program in nursing, with the clinical nurse specialist role at its core (see Table 6.1). The five-year curriculum plan is depicted in Table 6.2. In developing the plan, the group chose to use recommendations from the Institute of Medicine's (2003) report on health professions education as the organizing framework. (See Figure 6.1, p. 105.) Why is this clinical leadership role so timely?

- It moves the nursing profession away from years of divisive debate over entry into practice.
- It makes nursing more consistent with other health professions while also recognizing that multiple levels of providers still have value in the largest of the health professions, which is made up mostly of employees and often requires 24/7 operation.
- These nurses would work with a team of staff nurses in providing continuity of nursing care that is safer and more satisfying for patients and their families.
- These nurses would also be charged with being the retention officers of the future and with facilitating the transition of new graduates to the workplace.
- No new means of licensing/credentialing would be required beyond the existing legal recognition of the CNS.

(Text continued on p. 103).

TABLE 6.1   Curriculum Content Areas for Proposed Entry-Level Master's Program in Nursing

Patient-Centered Care

1. Basic clinical competence (by year 3)
   a. Assessment, planning, implementation, evaluation
   b. Prereq., A&P
   c. Basic fundamentals
   d. Pathophysiology and pharmacology
   e. Research-based practice
2. Advanced clinical competence (years 4 & 5)
   a. Advanced assessment
   b. Expertise beyond basic (guided clinical residency posteducation)
   c. Methodologies of care delivery
   d. Case management
3. Cultural/social care (general education/year 3 related to nursing)
   a. Understanding of impact of culture, psychosocial issues, and spirituality on health
   b. Alternative medicine
   c. Role and gender theory
   d. Diversity, language skills
4. Communication (general education and nursing thread)
   a. Personal insight and maturity
   b. Therapeutic communication skills
      i. Listening
      ii. Observation
   c. Communication styles
   d. Conflict management/resolution
   e. Crisis management
   f. Assertiveness skills
   g. Language mastery (oral and written)
   h. Negotiation skills
   i. Presentation skills
   j. Empathy
   k. Advocacy
   l. Intradisciplinary consultation
   m. Leading groups, public speaking (years 4 & 5)
5. Ethics (general education and nursing thread)
   a. Principles/models
   b. Social justice
   c. Ethical decision making
   d. Resource allocation
   e. Self-determination
   f. Advocacy
   g. Cultural considerations

TABLE 6.1 *(Continued)*

6. Teaching and learning (nursing thread)
   a. Learning styles of self and others
   b. Domains of learning
   c. Learning theory
   d. Age, culture, gender factors
   e. Coaching
   f. Outcome evaluation of learning
   g. Significant other inclusion in education
   h. Creating learning environment
   i. Identifying teaching moments
   j. Material development
   k. Community education
   l. Workplace education
   m. Adaptation
   n. Presentation skills (one-on-one and group)
   o. Being a lifelong learner
7. Resource management (years 4 & 5)
   a. Assessing patient and environment
   b. Fiscal responsibility
   c. Impact of staff turnover on care (staffing effectiveness)
   d. Ingenuity
      i. New product development
      ii. New care methods/modalities
   e. Benchmarking (hrs/pt/day)
      i. Ability to analyze
      ii. Evaluation of effect of resource management
   f. Resource allocation
      i. Material
      ii. Human
   g. Understanding reimbursement (payer and systems)
   h. Budgetary awareness
8. Critical thinking/decision making (nursing thread)
   a. Critical component of basic clinical competence
   b. Theory of critical thinking and decision making
   c. Application of process to all clinical situations
   d. Methodology of critical thinking
   e. Observation skill
9. Technology, genetics, other related (nursing thread)
   a. Basic use as related to patient care
   b. Lifelong learning
   c. Adaptation
   d. Time saving, improvement-evaluate effectiveness
   e. Effect on patient outcomes
   f. Professional accountability to be current
   g. Patient and family teaching

(continued)

TABLE 6.1   Curriculum Content Areas for Proposed Entry-Level Master's Program in Nursing *(Continued)*

Interdisciplinary Care
(Years 4 & 5 unless otherwise noted)

1. Collaboration
   a. Mutual respect/responsibility
   b. Mutual disagreement
   c. Valuing differences
   d. Consensus building
   i. Listening
      ii. Dialogue
      iii. Facilitation
      iv. Assertiveness
      v. Negotiation
   e. Teamwork (begin in year 3)
   f. Consultation
   g. Role theory
   h. Conflict management
   i. Self (year 3) and group assessment
      i. Professional socialization
      ii. Instruments of assessment
2. Communication
   a. Language proficiency (nonverbal, oral, written)
   b. Modalities of communication
      i. Public
      ii. Media
      iii. Political
      iv. Technology
         • PDA
         • Internet
         • Telehealth
   c. Crisis communication
   d. Groups (patients/families/colleagues/organizations)
   e. Professional culture
3. Healthcare finance/economics
   a. Cost benefit
   b. Present value
   c. Financial language
   d. Reimbursement/payer strategies
   e. Financial reporting/interpretation
   f. Return on investment
   g. Human resource management
   h. Material resource management
   i. Knowledge management (intellectual property)

TABLE 6.1   *(Continued)*

4. Clinical management/leadership
    a. Decision-making science
    b. Strategic planning
    c. Delegation/accountability
    d. Leadership theories
    e. Mentoring/precepting/coaching
    f. Care delivery models/staffing
    g. Case management
    h. Collaboration
    i. Clinical evaluation
    j. Team building
    k. Consultation
    l. Research-based innovation
5. Coordination and integration of care
    a. Health systems
        i. Micro
        ii. Macro
    b. Payer systems
    c. Cultural/social systems
    d. Resource procurement
    e. Referral systems
    f. Core competencies of all disciplines
    g. Oversight
        i. Licensure
        ii. Regulation
        iii. Certification
        iv. Accreditation
    h. Regulation and scopes of practice (begins in year 3)
    i. Labor law
6. Professional socialization (a–f in year 3)
    a. Professional image/behavior
    b. Responsibility to the profession
    c. Self-care
    d. Continued competence
    e. Code of ethics
    f. Communication
        i. Interdisciplinary
        ii. Peer
    g. Roles and responsibilities of advanced practice nurse
    h. Interdisciplinary residency

Informatics
(Years 4 & 5 unless otherwise noted)

1. Computer competence

(continued)

TABLE 6.1   Curriculum Content Areas for Proposed Entry-Level Master's Program in Nursing *(Continued)*

    a. Spreadsheets
    b. Field-specific technology
 2. Ethics and confidentiality of information
 3. Data management
    a. Entry
    b. Information sharing
 4. Statistical competence
 5. Globalization of information
 6. Judgment of data quality
 7. Distance intervention/telehealth
 8. PDA/Computerized entry
 9. Data-driven decision-making

Evidenced-Based Practice
(Year 4 & 5 unless otherwise noted)

 1. Theory (begins in year 2) from nursing and other disciplines
    a. Overall understanding of theory
    b. Understanding abstract thinking and how to think abstractly
    c. Value of other disciplines' theories to nursing and health care
 2. Research
    a. Methodology
    b. Statistics
    c. Quantitative vs. qualitative research
    d. Data collection
    e. Evaluation and application
    f. Implications of outcomes
    g. Assessing validity and reliability of research
       i. Refereed vs. nonrefereed
 3. Causation vs. correlation
 4. Participation in collaborative research
 5. Grant writing
 6. Best practices, standards
 7. Assimilation of new knowledge
 8. Dissemination of information
    a. Writing for publication
    b. Oral presentation
    c. Journal clubs
 9. Integration of research from other disciplines
10. Utilizing research techniques
    a. Existing data
    b. Available resources
       i. Human
      ii. Material
     iii. Fiscal

TABLE 6.1   *(Continued)*

Quality Improvement
(Year 4 & 5 unless otherwise noted)

1. Decisions based on continuous feedback loop
2. Structure, Process, Outcomes
   a. Health
   b. Cost effectiveness
   c. Satisfaction
3. Best practices/delivery models
4. Benchmarking
5. Systems focus
6. Strategic management/planning
7. Outcome reporting
8. Regulation and health policy
9. Employer of choice designation/workplace excellence

EXEMPLAR #2—DEVELOPING A STATEWIDE ARTICULATION MODEL: THE SOUTH CAROLINA EXPERIENCE

The South Carolina Colleagues in Caring Project (SCCIC) began intensive data collection upon being funded in 1997. The data clearly showed that the state was facing a shortage of registered nurses that would progressively worsen through 2015. A closer look at the data revealed that:

- 68% of doctorally prepared nurses were over the age of 50, and 29% were over the age of 60
- 38% of master's-prepared nurses were over the age of 50
- 65% of all licensed nurses had less than a baccalaureate degree in nursing
- the average age of registered nurses in the state was 45 years
- the numbers of LPNs and RNs returning to school to advance their nursing education had diminished each year over the previous five years

It was evident from the data that it was time to take action to rapidly increase the number of nurses with advanced degrees as well as increase the supply of registered nurses. Educators representing every nursing program in the state were invited to a "visioning

TABLE 6.2   Five-Year Curriculum Plan

Years 1 and 2
    Anatomy and Physiology (2 semesters)
    Chemistry: organic/inorganic (1 semester)
    Microbiology
    English (2 semesters)
    Spanish (2 semesters)*
    Psychology: Human Development Across Life Span
    Sociology: World Cultures
    Mathematics*/Statistics
    Computer Science*
    Economics
    Philosophy/Ethics
    Nutrition
    Physical Education
    Electives (2)
    Seminar course: Dimensions of Professional Nursing

Year 3
    Health Appraisal of Individual, Family, and Community
    Professional Nursing Foundation
    Patient-Centered Culturally Competent Care
    Integrated prelicensure content, mostly CAI, with some didactic and
        clinical hours, leading to successful passing of NCLEX-RN

Year 4
    Advanced Pathophysiology
    Advanced Pharmacology
    Advanced diagnostic reasoning/methods/tools
    Interdisciplinary care
    Informatics

Year 5
    Care delivery methodologies
    Evidence-based care
    Quality improvement
    Internship/residency final semester, culminating in awarding of MSN

Postgraduation
  • Continue residency to meet clinical requirements, leading to CNS
    certification
  • Complete post-master's NP certificate program
  • Complete additional requirements for nursing administration (MBA)
  • Complete additional coursework in curriculum, evaluation, and
    teaching methods for nursing education

*May advance place/place out.

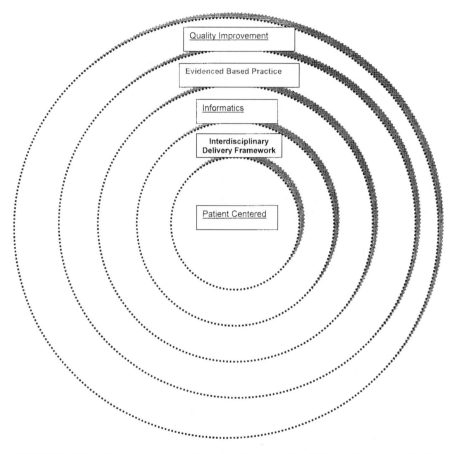

FIGURE 6.1   Concepts from the Institute of Medicine's Framework for Health Professions Education.

retreat" in fall 1999 to formulate a plan to address the critical issues facing the profession. By the conclusion of the retreat, a document delineating the mission, purpose, scope, and value of each level of nursing education was developed. This document, entitled *A Model for Differentiated Entry Level Nursing Practice by Educational Program Type*© would serve as a basis for the future development of the South Carolina Articulation Model.

History of Articulation in South Carolina

In 1995 the South Carolina Statewide Task Force on Nursing Transfer and Articulation presented a report to the South Carolina Commission on Higher Education that established guidelines to facilitate the progression of students in good standing who needed to transfer from one South Carolina public associate degree in nursing or bachelor of science degree in nursing program to another. The guidelines established the criteria for eligibility and the mechanism for transfer of both nursing and general education courses.

In addition, guidelines were developed to facilitate progression of registered nurses who graduated from a South Carolina public NLNAC (National League for Nursing Accrediting Commission)-accredited ADN program to a public BSN program. Eligibility criteria and a transfer mechanism were defined that provided a minimum of 60 semester hours of credit (nursing and general education combined) to be awarded by the receiving institution if all criteria were met.

The agreement also recommended a public ADN program would adopt a maximum of 68 semester credit hours and a public BSN program would adopt a maximum of 128 semester credit hours. The South Carolina Commission on Higher Education approved the model and required implementation by fall 1997 for all public ADN and BSN programs. The commission charged the South Carolina Council of Deans and Directors of Nursing Education Programs with the responsibility for reviewing and monitoring the outcomes of the transfer model and to report to the commission at five-year intervals.

While the agreement addressed some of the issues of interinstitutional transfer as well as offered a basis for some standardization in curricula by capping the number of credit hours by type of program, there were several areas that were not addressed in the plan. Licensed practical nursing programs were not addressed in the transfer model. In addition, there was some confusion on the part of educational faculty regarding the process for validation of prior coursework. The South Carolina Council of Deans and Directors agreed to work with the SCCIC in evaluating the effectiveness of the present model and building on this model to accomplish the goal of formulating a comprehensive statewide model for articulation.

The SCCIC applied to the Helene Fuld Health Trust for a grant to develop a statewide system of nursing articulation. The grant was funded in January 2000, and the articulation project began.

Process

To facilitate a common understanding of articulation and its implications for nursing education, an expert consultant was retained. Dr. Mary Fry Rapson, RN, Project Director of the National Colleagues in

Caring Project, provided consultation and facilitation skills to assist the conference participants to gain consensus on the model and shared her expertise on designing statewide articulation models. An educational mobility steering committee was appointed to guide the work of the project.

Representatives from each nursing education program in South Carolina, along with leaders from a variety of nursing practice settings met together in three statewide conferences over a period of one year to conceptualize the model. In the first conference Dr. Rapson presented extensive information on the politics of articulation, reviewed terminology related to articulation, compared advantages and disadvantages of selected validation mechanisms, and took the participants through the process for developing an articulation model.

Prior to the first conference, several focus groups were conducted across the state with currently enrolled RN-BSN students and recent LPN-ADN and RN-BSN graduates; currently practicing LPNs, Diploma, and ADNs; and employers. Dr. Jan Bellack, RN, FAAN, (Co-Project Director of the SCCIC) presented the results from the focus groups and summarized the themes with relevance for nurse educators, for employers/practice settings, and the general findings and themes (see Table 6.3).

The results of an articulation survey—reflecting the current status of articulation in the state's practical nursing, associate degree nursing, and bachelor degree nursing programs—were also disseminated to the conference participants. Dialogue in small- and large-group sessions provided the educational mobility steering committee with information to devise a draft for a proposed articulation model to discuss at the second conference.

Articulation Model Development

The goal of the educational mobility steering committee was to draft an articulation model that would provide two options: an "institutional validation," or direct transfer of credits for students who met specific criteria as stated in the model, and an option for "individual validation" for students who did not meet the specific criteria but could receive credit through a validation process determined by the admitting institution. The challenge was to develop criteria for institutional validation that would be acceptable to all the educational programs as well as legally acceptable to the board of nursing, the accreditation organizations, and the state educational oversight commissions.

TABLE 6.3   Themes Derived from Focus Groups

Themes with Relevance for Nurse Educators
- Give credit for current knowledge or competency.
- Adjust inflexible prerequisites and grade point average requirements.
- Establish common core of prerequisites.
- Schedule courses well in advance.
- Provide more options and flexibility in course scheduling.
- Use customer friendly and knowledgeable frontline contacts in schools.
- Minimize changes in program and course requirements.
- Provide information about scholarships and other financial aid.

Themes with Relevance to Employers/Practice Settings
- Provide tuition assistance as a benefit.
- Provide release time to attend classes, flexible scheduling, differential recognition upon completion.

General Findings/Themes
- Those who pursue educational mobility do so largely because it is a personal goal or ambition.
- Value is added by BSN education: community perspective, professional issues, political involvement, teamwork, inquiry, evidence-based practice, patient advocacy, and liberal education.

The steering committee drafted a set of assumptions to guide their work. Table 6.4 delineates the assumptions that were approved by the participants during the second conference. Questions raised during development of the draft model included areas such as

- how to address students that graduated from non-NLNAC accredited programs
- how to deal with students from out-of-state programs
- whether there should be a work requirement
- how long after graduation courses are still acceptable for direct transfer
- how the LPN-RN student will be evaluated

Tables 6.5 and 6.6 provide an overview of the basic criteria established for both institutional and individual validation for the RN-BSN articulation model and the LPN-RN model.

The draft of the proposed statewide articulation model was the focus of discussion during the second statewide nurse educator conference. While most of the proposed model was received very positively, there was continued discussion about the newly formulated

TABLE 6.4   Assumptions Underlying the South Carolina Statewide Articulation Model

An effective articulation model must protect the quality and integrity of both sending and accepting institutions and also provide fair, equitable access to undergraduate nursing education for registered nurses and licensed practical nurses. The following assumptions for the South Carolina Statewide Articulation Model were synthesized from several sources, including discussions during statewide conferences, the nursing literature, and previously designed articulation models in other states.

1. All nursing education programs have worth and are valuable.
2. Each type of nursing education program uses a core of nursing knowledge, skills, abilities, and values on which to build. *The South Carolina Model for Differentiated Nursing Practice by Educational Program Type©* is the conceptual framework on which the South Carolina Statewide Articulation Model is designed.
3. The South Carolina Statewide Articulation Model builds on the South Carolina Articulation and Transfer Agreement established in 1995 and approved by the South Carolina Commission on Higher Education.
4. Articulation in nursing education is intended to minimize duplication of efforts and to reduce students' time and costs in advancing their nursing education.
5. All South Carolina public nursing education programs will comply with the statewide articulation model.
6. All educational institutions have the right to establish their own unique mission, goals, and standards for admission, progression, and graduation.
7. The demand for nurses with increased educational preparation is growing and forcing nursing education to change to a system that facilitates upward mobility and life-long learning in nursing education.
8. The progression to the next level of nursing is self-determined and based on the nurse's desire and abilities.

Source: Loquist, R., and Brady, M., *South Carolina Statewide Articulation Model,* May 2001 (p. 7).

LPN-RN articulation criteria. Based on the discussion, two task forces were convened to explore the issue of whether LPN programs should operate under a cap on credit hours as the RN programs did, and the second task force was to address the issue of developing a statewide LPN-RN transition course with core content delineated. The first issue of capping credits for LPN programs was important to the participants because the range in credit hours for LPN programs across the state was from 38 to 58 semester hours. The

TABLE 6.5   South Carolina RN-BSN Articulation Model

Requirements of the 1995 Statewide Nursing Transfer and Articulation Guide

1. Associate degree nursing (AND) programs in South Carolina public institutions shall adopt a maximum of 68 semester credit hour ADN degree.

2. BSN programs in South Carolina public institutions shall adopt a maximum of 128 semester credit hour BSN degree.

3. A minimum of 60 credits of college transfer general education and nursing course credit taken at any in-state NLNAC accredited ADN-granting institution will transfer and apply toward a BSN degree at any in-state public institution offering the BSN degree.

4. Recommendations on ADN to ADN and BSN to BSN transfer should be continued and updated to reflect current courses.

5. Private in-state institutions may adopt these requirements as desired.

RN to BSN articulation Option 1 Direct transfer	RN to BSN articulation Option 2 Individual validation
A minimum of 25 semester hours of nursing credits will be awarded by the receiving institution without educational mobility testing or validation if the applicant meets the following criteria: • Graduate from an NLNAC accredited, credit-bearing program • Has a current, active South Carolina license • Meets admission requirements of receiving institution • Meets residency requirements of receiving institution	Individual validation of credit awarded will be determined by the receiving institution if the applicant is a: • Graduate from a non-NLNAC accredited program • Graduate from a noncredit-bearing program A minimum of 25 semester hours of nursing credits will be awarded upon completion of validation if the applicant meets the following criteria: • Has a current, active South Carolina license • Meets admission requirements of receiving institution • Meets residency requirements of receiving institution

TABLE 6.5 *(Continued)*

Non-nursing transfer credit:	Non-nursing transfer credit:
• General education courses listed in the Statewide Articulation Agreement as transferable from state technical colleges to public senior institutions will be transferred directly. • General education courses completed from out-of-state institutions may transfer subject to individual school policies.	• General education courses listed in the Statewide Articulation Agreement as transferable from state technical colleges to public senior institutions ill be transferred directly. • General education courses completed from out-of-state institutions may transfer subject to individual school policies.

ADN programs were already capped at 68 semester hours and BSN programs at 128 semester hours. Conceivably, a student graduating from the 58-credit hour LPN program who received no credit for prior learning could spend 126 semester hours earning an associate degree in nursing. This was seen as a serious problem and counter-productive to increasing the number of LPNs seeking advanced degrees.

During the third statewide nurse educator conference, the proposed articulation plan was approved with very few amendments. The participants voted to recommend capping the LPN programs at 48 semester hours and providing for 15 semester hours of nursing credit to be awarded by direct transfer for students meeting the specific criteria delineated in the model. RN-BSN students would receive 25 semester hours of nursing credit if they met the specific criteria in the model. An educational pathway was developed to provide a quick overview of the model (see Figure 6.2).

Following the three conferences, the proposed model was presented to the South Carolina Council of Deans and Directors for acceptance. The commission on higher education received the model during a commission meeting in November 2001 and approved its implementation as a mandatory model for the state's nursing education programs. The commission further provided that the South Carolina Board of Nursing monitor compliance with the model. The State Board of Nursing also received and accepted the model for statewide implementation.

TABLE 6.6   South Carolina LPN to ADN Articulation Model

1. LPN programs located in the state's technical colleges shall adopt a maximum of 48 semester hours credit for a diploma in practical nursing by fall 2003.
2. LPN programs located in the state's technical colleges shall adopt a maximum of 31 semester hours of nursing credit by fall 2003.
3. LPN programs located in the state's technical colleges are strongly encouraged to adopt general education courses that are listed in the Statewide Articulation Agreement.
4. LPN programs in the state's career and technology centers shall review their curricula and reach consensus on an acceptable range of maximum clock hours for a practical nursing diploma.
5. LPN programs in the state's career and technology centers are strongly encouraged to collaborate with technical colleges to offer general education courses that are transferable to the technical college system.
6. LPN-ADN applicants must meet the admission and progression requirements of the receiving institution to include a three-semester hour credit LPN-ADN transition course that reflects the recommended core content and learning activities as follows:
   - Core content:
     A. Communication
     B. Roles: Provider of care, manager of care, member of the discipline, patient educator
     C. Ethical/Legal principles
     D. Critical thinking concepts
     E. Nursing process: Assessment, analysis, planning, implementation, evaluation
   - Core learning activities to promote student success:
     A. Written assignments
     B. Multiple-choice tests
     C. Case study with plan of care
   - Skills validation for the LPN-ADN student may be accomplished through the transition course or through successful completion of the first clinical nursing course in the ADN program.

LPN to ADN articulation Option 1 Direct transfer	LPN to ADN articulation Option 2 Individual validation
A minimum of 15 semester hours of nursing credits will be awarded without educational mobility testing or validation if the applicant meets the following criteria:	Individual validation of credit awarded will be determined by the receiving institution if the applicant: • Graduated from a non-NLNAC accredited program

TABLE 6.6 *(Continued)*

LPN to ADN articulation Option 1 Direct transfer	LPN to ADN articulation Option 2 Individual validation
• Graduates from an NLNAC-accredited, credit-bearing program • Has a current, active South Carolina LPN license • Meets admission and progression requirements of receiving institution • Meets residency requirements of receiving institution	• Graduated from a noncredit-bearing program A minimum of 15 semester hours of nursing credits will be awarded upon completion of validation if the applicant meets the following criteria: • Has a current, active South Carolina license • Meets admission requirements of receiving institution • Meets residency requirements of receiving institution
Non-nursing transfer credit: • General education courses listed in the Statewide Articulation Agreement as transferable from state technical colleges to public senior institutions will be transferred directly. • General education courses completed from out-of-state institutions may transfer subject to individual school policies.	*Non-nursing transfer credit:* • General education courses listed in the Statewide Articulation Agreement as transferable from state technical colleges to public senior institutions ill be transferred directly. • General education courses completed from out-of-state institutions may transfer subject to individual school policies.

Summary

While development of the statewide articulation model was the primary focus of the statewide nurse educators' conferences, there were numerous benefits that emerged from the project. This was the first time that educators from all levels of nursing education and employers from various practice settings were able to meet in a single forum for dialogue. The LPN educators particularly were grateful for the opportunity to be seen as peers and to have input into the process.

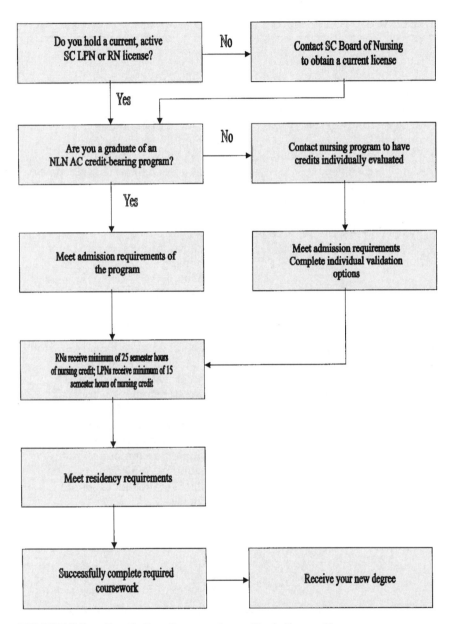

FIGURE 6.2   South Carolina nursing articulation pathway.

Numerous casual conversations during time for networking resulted in collaboration among programs to initiate joint Internet-based nursing courses and other creative programming. Accelerated curricula such as LPN-BSN and RN-MSN were explored and later initiated. There was a new foundation for collaboration formed that continue to benefit the students and employers who are desperately trying to fill nursing positions with appropriately educated staff.

Early evaluation reveals that implementation of the South Carolina articulation model has increased the number of students seeking advanced education in nursing in the state. Employers have become more aggressive in offering financial support and flexible schedules to assist students to return to school for advanced degrees. The current challenge is to prepare sufficient faculty to increase the educational capacity needed to deal with the success of generating interest in nursing as a career and advanced education for practicing nurses.

EXEMPLAR #3—ELECTRONIC LEARNING IN TEXAS: ACCESS AND QUALITY

A revolution in higher learning is underway. Revolutions in higher education are not new; the present-day collective changes and improvements in the academy are viewed as the third major evolution in the presentation and organization of content for learning (Ehrmann, 1999). Early organized learning concentrated on explaining and conversation, usually with a tutor teaching small groups or one person, e.g., Socrates. The first revolution occurred as reading and writing skills spread deeper through the classes in the population. The advent of the printing press escalated the availability of written materials for use by the ordinary person. These events laid the foundation for enormous increases in the scale of education, albeit at a cost of increased distance between the learner and the teacher. Almost 2,000 years later, the second revolution took place with the concentration of scattered scholars, learners, and academic resources into a community where they could interact spontaneously—the campus environment. Access was increased for some, whereas others were shut out again due to increased distance from the center of learning. Now we are in the midst of the third revolution: The Internet is the driving force for this evolution of higher learning. The Internet provides the opportunity to "have it all"—two-way communication, rich media content, and ready access to historical and current print resources. The issue of distance is no longer an inhibiting factor preventing educational access and availability. The Internet revolution offers substantial improvements in both availability and access, allowing consumer choice, and demand appears to drive the assurance of quality.

Nursing has consistently sought to provide access to degree and continuing education programs with varying levels of success. Often the transmission medium prohibited quality transmission of the content, and both availability and access have been especially difficult in some of the outlying geographical areas of the country. The Internet revolution offers solutions to these issues and, for the first time, truly enables learning, anytime, anywhere—unencumbered by time and place. Technology and distributed learning opportunities are now able to be seamlessly integrated and provided in a high-tech and high-touch environment. Barriers now are grounded in attitudes and cultures that view change and reorganization as variables to be prevented. Yet clearly, the demand for education is being driven by elements in our society as never before. The high school diploma no longer is a guarantee of a reasonable, life-long income. The entry-level standard is moving rapidly to the baccalaureate degree, presenting an imperative to the academy to inculcate the technology and meet the needs of the population. Innovators and early adopters incorporating enabling technology have always abounded in the discipline of nursing, and thus spreading the Internet through our curricula by reforming access and availability will take place rapidly.

Electronic Learning in Nursing Education (eLine) is a seamless, articulated, collaborative delivery system for entry-level nursing curricula and is available anytime, anywhere. It is based in the nursing school at Texas A&M University—Corpus Christi and Del Mar College. Using a competency-based, self-paced modular breakdown of existing associate- and baccalaureate-degree curricula that meet all essential standards and accreditation requirements, eLine solves the quality, availability, and access issues. It is a truly innovative solution that offers the possibility to enroll 10,000 new students within three years when the system becomes fully operational in the fall of 2004.

The U.S. Bureau of Labor Statistics predicts 1 million available positions for registered nurses in 2010 (Bureau of Labor Statistics, 2004). Given the present rate of graduation from all entry-level programs and factoring in predicted retirements, approximately half of the 1 million positions will not be able to be filled. This growth in need exceeds 21% compared to a collective job growth of 14% in all other professions. The National League for Nursing (2003) projects waiting lists in excess of 30,000 students for all entry-level programs, diploma, associate, and baccalaureate degrees. The American Association of Colleges of Nursing (AACN) report 15,944 qualified students were denied entry to baccalaureate programs in the last academic year (AACN, 2004). The nursing professoriate is aging (average age of 51), and nurses are not entering the faculty ranks as rapidly as needed to make up the current shortfall, much less meet future needs (AACN, 2003). Frequently, new doctoral graduates already have a faculty position or are recruited into positions other than teaching. Figuring in the predicted retirements yields approximately 100 net new faculty by 2010. We must find truly innovative ways to address these issues, or the provision of high-quality, cost-effective care will decline rapidly, injuring the public's health and well-being and triggering long-term, irreversible consequences.

When there are not enough nurses, patient safety is threatened and health care quality is diminished. The Institute of Medicine's landmark report of 1999 estimated that between 44,000 and 98,000 people die each year as a result of errors in the health care delivery system—more that those who die in motor vehicle accidents, from breast cancer, or from AIDS and equaling the number of deaths from a 747 airplane crashing every day for one year (Institute of Medicine, 2000)

Among the problems that commonly occur are adverse medication events and improper transfusions, surgical injuries and wrong-site surgery, suicides, restraint-related injuries or death, falls, burns, pressure ulcers, and mistaken patient identities. Nurses who are caring for far too many patients or working too many hours struggle to intercept 86% of the medication errors made by others before such errors reach the patient. Needleman, Buerhaus, Mattke, Stewart, and Zelevinsky (2002) reported that better care for hospitalized patients (N = 6,180,628), as evidenced by shorter length of stay and lower rates of urinary tract infections, upper gastrointestinal bleeding, pneumonia, and shock or cardiac arrest, resulted from a higher proportion of hours of nursing care provided by registered nurses and a greater number of hours of care by registered nurses per day. A cross-sectional analysis of the outcomes data found that surgical patients experienced lower mortality when care was provided by baccalaureate-prepared registered nurses versus less-prepared caregivers (N = 232,342).

The classic on-campus classroom/patient room dyad model cannot meet the demand for the nurses needed to provide for the health of the population. More students cannot be admitted to already full programs. Yet we know that the current curricula produce nurses educated to provide optimal care. Solutions lie in establishing more pathways to make the nursing curricula available to students.

The eLine Partnership invested in substantial study of the future needs of the Greater Coastal Bend region of south Texas as well as looking across the country for similarities in need for the composition and capacity of the registered nurse workforce to provide for the health needs of the population in the future. (See Table 6.7.) With over $7 million from numerous funding sources, as listed in Table 6.8, the fully online entry-level delivery system for associate and baccalaureate degrees was created. The eLine Partnership is a collaborative anchored by the nursing faculty at Texas A&M University—Corpus Christi and Del Mar College. Other key stakeholders in the regional community and at national levels have been members of the partnership where their contributions were relevant to the specific initiative underway. Key long-term partners include the Coastal Bend Health Education Center and the South Texas Public Broadcast System. All of the regional health care delivery systems have participated in the Partnership and are part of the planning phase for the next steps in this long-term project addressing nursing education. In addition, the business community is a contributor, both fiscally and through active team member participation. Foundations as evident in Table 6.8 have been key support partners, enabling the overall initiative to continue moving forward. Regulatory oversight is provided by both the Texas Board of Nurse Examiners and the Texas Higher Education Coordinating Board.

ELine is a needed alternative access point for entry-level nursing education. It is the online, competency-based, modular delivery system for existing curricula at the ADN and BSN levels. Building from the competencies as organized by the Board of Nurse Examiners for the State of Texas and based on work done by the National League of Nurses and the Association of American Colleges of Nurses, the curricula of the associate degree in nursing program at Del Mar College and the baccalaureate nursing program at Texas A&M University—Corpus Christi were "unpacked" into 107 competency-based modules. These modules have been "repacked" into the individual courses at each school. When the student registers for a course online, the modules for that course open and the student may progress at his or her own pace, taking up to one year to complete the total modules for the course. The modules are significantly

TABLE 6.7   Participants in eLine Partnership, 2004

Texas A&M University—Corpus Christi
Del Mar College
Coastal Bend Health Education Center
Public Broadcasting System of South Texas
Colleagues in Caring Network, a project of The Robert Wood Johnson
    Foundation

TABLE 6.8   Funding Support for eLine Partnership, 2004

Learning Anywhere, Anytime Program

The Robert Wood Johnson Foundation

Fund for the Improvement of Post Secondary Education, United States
   Department of Education

Texas Public Broadcasting Educational Network

Telecommunications Infrastructure Fund Board

Public Broadcasting System of South Texas

Texas A&M University—Corpus Christi

Del Mar College

Coastal Bend Health Education Network

smaller repositories of content than traditional semester-based courses, but all the requisite material is present when the relevant course modules are complete. Completed modules are credited to the relevant course shells, and when the courses are complete the grade is posted to the transcript. The modular format allows for smooth transition from the ADN to the BSN with no repetition of content.

Students apply for admission online and are able to complete the registration and payment process online, as well as purchase books and other needed supplies. Virtually all services are available to them online as is the entire undergraduate general education core curriculum. Course registration is available online every five weeks; students are not bound by semester or location. The eLine students have a dedicated advisor who holds a master's degree in nursing and is very technology proficient. Screening processes are contained in the Webspace to help students decide if online nursing education will indeed meet their needs. Numerous support services are available through the library

The eLine delivery system includes the didactic portion of 10 clinical modules; the clinical modules in eLine are listed in Table 6.9. As with the other modules, the clinical modules incorporate the specific elements required by the degree programs and meet state and accrediting requirements. Clinical experiences for the eLine delivery system are both degree based and specific to the student's individualized progress through the nursing program. Students work with appropriately credentialed preceptors and faculty, both full time and associate, in the health care delivery system. Two large health care delivery systems are founding partners, the CHRISTUS Health System and Texas Health Resources. These two systems

TABLE 6.9   eLine Clinical Modules

Health Assessment Clinical
Clinical Care of Children and Families
Community Health Clinical
Clinical Care of Parents, Newborns, and Women
Coordination of Care Clinical
Clinical Care of the Adult Patient I
Clinical Care of the Adult Patient II
Clinical Care of Adult Patients III
Clinical Care of Adult Patients IV
Clinical Care of Mental Health Patients

contain 75 institutions in five states that are used on a regional basis for clinical learning experiences. As enrollment expands, other health care delivery organizations will be solicited as partners. They will provide select members of their staff to act in the clinical adjunct preceptor or faculty role for the eLine students. The clinical adjunct faculty and preceptors meet all education and credentialing requirements in the relevant state and accreditation requirements for the affiliated nursing program site.

Proposals are in review at three agencies as this chapter is being written. These initiatives propose the eLine Faculty Alliance. The Alliance will be an innovative configuration of faculty and nursing programs across the country for nationwide, large-scale delivery of eLine. Sufficient fully qualified part-time faculty will be sought, one per module (for 107 modules at this writing), enabling large-scale enrollment into the program. Associate- and baccalaureate-degree nursing programs will be invited to join the Alliance and to deliver their curricula via the modular format. The modules have been created so that rebranding and reconfiguration into different curriculum patterns is possible. In addition, a national advisory board will be created to provide oversight with various issues that will inevitably arise due to the uniqueness of both state regulations and nursing programs in higher education.

Nursing education is at a crossroads. We entered into the campus revolution of higher education and adapted our apprenticeship system to one of lecture halls and on-campus learning laboratories. This model has served us well. We have, over time, created the best nursing education curriculum in the world, as demonstrated time and again through numerous research studies. We know this by the constant invitations from other countries to our schools and colleges of nursing to help build their nursing education programs. However, if we are unable to meet the entry demand and create and retain faculty, nursing may not survive. Is that the next revolution for this discipline?

EXEMPLAR #4—VERMONT NURSE INTERNSHIP PROJECT: TRANSITION TO PRACTICE MODEL

The Vermont Nurse Internship Project (VNIP) is a transition model that has proven its worth. The project that was undertaken in response to the looming staffing issues identified in 1999 by the Vermont Organization of Nurse Leaders (VONL). VONL partnered with the Vermont Association of Hospitals and Health Systems (VAHHS) to commission research on nursing workforce issues specific to Vermont. The resulting report, the *Vermont Nursing Report* became the basis for further collaborative work and strategic planning relating to the pending workforce crisis. Six strategic goals for dealing with the crisis were identified in the report, available online (http://www.vahhs.org/lucie/Vonl/VONL%20Presentation.htm). Two of these goals became the focus of the internship project:

V. Create a formal nursing internship program that provides adequate practical clinical experience for novice nurses to function at a competent level when they enter the work force. This would force a marriage of schools of nursing and fields of practice that could strengthen both institutions, while promoting the preparation of nurses able to handle the currently complex and demanding field of health care.
VI. Expand clinical opportunities for students by increasing the use of clinical staff as preceptors in specialty areas.

Grant funding was obtained to support a half-time director's position to lead development and implementation of the model/project, and the Vermont Nurse Internship Project (VNIP) was established.

Model Development and Implementation

At the initial VNIP meeting, it was determined that three levels of internship were needed: (1) a student extern program for expanded undergraduate clinical experience; (2) a transition to practice internship following graduation to provide an organized, supportive transition to practice that included educational support, competency development, and skills evaluation; and (3) specialty care internships to provide the extensive additional education and support for work in a specialty care area such as surgery, intensive care, home care, long-term care, etc. Initial model development targeted new graduate RNs and transition to practice. It was decided that the internship would be based on a precepted delivery model. As a result, two programs were developed, one for the interns (new graduates) and another for the development and support of clinical staff preceptors.

Unique aspects of this project include the collaborative workgroup composed of nurse leaders from practice settings, academia, and the board of nursing and the focus on a model configuration that can be applied statewide and across the continuum of care. The internship model used Lenburg's competency outcomes performance assessment model (Lenburg, 1999) for the core outline of the RN role and competency-based skills verification. The specific subskills for each of Lenburg's eight core practice competencies were identified with input from all practice areas to establish a competency verification form that outlined the core role of the generalist RN in most, if not all, direct care settings. The initial form was used in the first pilot during the summer of 2000. Based on outcomes data and feedback from educators and preceptors using the model in the pilot, it was modified and then underwent a second pilot during 2001. Thus the model and its components were validated as a standardized model for delivery in multiple settings. The model was found to provide structure for experiential learning that can address the needs of the new graduate, specialty care internships, and/or the clinical component of a reentry program.

The initial outcomes analysis resulted in recognizing the urgent need for added preparation for preceptors. A preceptor development focus group that included the directors of three of the state's nursing programs convened. They assisted in shifting this essential preparation into theory and research-based education that is delivered via an independent learning module and two days of workshop presentation. This initial education totals 18.6 contact hours of interactive teaching/learning. Thanks to a partnership with grant-funded specialty care internships, we have been able to offer this standardized education to direct care providers from all regions and specialties within the state. The preceptor workshops have offered an ideal venue for collecting demographic data on these clinical experts so that we can identify those who might be interested in a future teaching role.

The statewide, standardized approach to preceptor development is another unique aspect of this project. It has led to development of a credentialing process for preceptors. This credentialing offers recognition and reward for this key teaching/support role, while establishing a pool of clinical preceptors who have all had the same educational preparation, support, and skills development/evaluation.

The internship has been in place as an active educational process since 2000 and has seen annual growth and expansion. Its impact has expanded through collaboration with various non-Vermont health care agencies who request consulting time and model adoption. The project currently has grant funding that will strengthen the VNIP coalition, expand implementation at additional sites/settings, develop the model for use in home care and public health settings, continue and/or expand preceptor development, and collect data specific to nurse retention in rural and/or medically underserved areas. The National Council of State Boards of Nursing (NCSBN) is finalizing plans for a research project that will be done collaboratively with the VNIP to evaluate both program outcomes and differences in clinical practice resulting from the model.

Internship Model

The internship is a formal, postlicensure educational program designed to extend the basic nurse education preparation, proficiency, and skills of new graduate and transitioning nurses. Each intern has completed a guided course of nursing education. The internship curriculum is designed to give experience and repeated practice application to demonstrate successful transition of this learning into the specific clinical practice setting. It includes individual studies, staff development courses, clinical conferences, and one-on-one support and instruction from a preceptor. The purpose of the internship is to advance clinical practice skills needed to deliver safe, comprehensive care in existing and emerging organized health care systems.

An internship session may include up to five preceptor/intern teams starting at the same time and lasting 10 weeks. At least 40 hours are devoted to didactic components within the program, and required content topics include, but are not limited to, standards of care, managed care, cultural competence, quality improvement, IV access/therapy, medication administration, and pain management. Interns are not considered as part of the staffing mix, and each is paired with a qualified preceptor. The patients assigned to interns will also be part of their preceptor's assignment, and preceptors progressively allocate patient care activities to the intern. The preceptors act as mentors and role models, leading the intern through his or her daily clinical experiences on the unit. On a weekly basis, the intern and the preceptor, and/or clinical educator will meet to establish/evaluate goals and work with critical thinking skills. Delivery of the internship requires release time for support of educational preparation, didactic instruction, goal setting, weekly conference, and support group meetings—approximately 200 hours of educator time for each internship session.

Competencies

The internship provides practice and verification of competencies that are based on the competency outcomes performance assessment model (Lenburg, 1999). The internship's competency verification form delineates specific criteria that address Lenburg's essential skills of assessment and interventions, communications, critical thinking, human caring/relationships, management, leadership, teaching, and knowledge integration.

Roles and Responsibilities Required to Support the Model

The clinical educator directs the facility-specific internship, provides didactic sessions for the intern, and offers ongoing support and resources for the preceptor/intern team. The preceptor develops learning goals/objectives in collaboration with the intern and clinical educator, assesses the intern's experience level and learning style, and plans learning experiences accordingly. He/she is responsible for choosing the patient assignment based on educational goals and objectives and sharing that assignment by progressively assigning patient care responsibilities to the intern. Along with planning, the preceptor provides daily feedback to the intern and collaborates with the clinical educator and nurse manager to evaluate progress and address issues. The intern is responsible for active participation in all components of the internship and completion of documentation.

Early Outcomes

- A 2000 satisfaction survey showed a greater than 40% improvement in satisfaction with transition to practice and new graduate competency.
- For the initial pilot, 49% of the nurse interns came from out of state residence or attended schools.
- Retention data from tertiary care center—Retention of those who completed orientation in 1999 was 75%, whereas new graduates who completed an internship showed a 93% retention rate for each of the following two years.

- Position vacancy rate—At one participating agency, the medical/surgical unit had suffered an unrelenting vacancy rate of 20%. This agency credits the internship/preceptor program with the current vacancy rate of 0% for the entire nursing department. This hospital now has no recruitment or position advertising costs for nursing positions.

Preceptor Program

The preceptor training and credentialing program is developed for nursing staff who work with graduate nurses, students, or new hires, or who cross train of staff. Development of this education and support has a two-fold purpose. The first expected outcome is that precepting RNs will improve their skills in teaching, coaching, mentoring, leadership, communication, and evaluation. Thus they can effectively work with nursing interns to help them gain competencies expected within the internship and outlined on a competency checklist. The second expected outcome is a change in the culture of the work environment. The program supports a transition from the current crisis-driven—and intimidating and isolating—workplace to a more supportive environment designed to assist the transition of a novice nurse into successful practice. This program is designed to build capacity both in individuals and in the environment. It will foster development of leadership skills and professionalism at a grass-roots level.

Preceptor Competencies

During the internship experience, the preceptor demonstrates effective skills in teaching techniques; listening, observational, and feedback techniques; design and planning experiences to operationalize the competency checklist in the clinical practice setting; evaluation and provision of constructive criticism and praise of achievements; minimization of reality shock; facilitation of conflict resolution; assistance to the intern in setting daily goals and plans; and encouragement, coaching, and motivation skill sets.

The clinical educator will be responsible for supporting the preceptor working to attain these skills and will validate that the skills are demonstrated with competence. The preceptor program is a formal, postlicensure educational program designed to increase knowledge, teaching, and communication skills of experienced nurses. These educational workshops are also used by specialty care area personnel for continued development of experienced staff in surgery, intensive care, psychiatric, and other special care areas.

While providing additional educational resources, this joint effort benefits the internship project by moving the workplace culture farther toward support of the novice/advanced beginner. We currently offer six workshops per year and accept a maximum of 30 participants per two-day offering.

The research- and theory-based course curriculum addresses role/responsibilities of the preceptor/intern, stages of Benner's model of novice to expert (Benner, 1984), principles of teaching/learning, learning styles, delegation/legal implications, team building, personality style, effective communication techniques, conflict management, generational issues, competence of new RNs in clinical practice, promoting critical thinking in the novice, and issues/concerns related to precepting.

Preceptor Credentialing Program

The preceptor training and credentialing program was developed for RN staff members who meet credentialing requirements. This program recognizes and rewards Vermont nurse preceptors through validation of their dedicated commitment to teaching and mentoring colleagues and novices. Application requirements include clinical practice hours, basic and ongoing education specific to the role, verification of precepting at a proficient level of practice, references, and résumé submission.

Recommendations

Along with investing in transition programs for new graduates, our healthcare systems need to ensure the development and support of preceptors in the clinical setting. Most of today's transition programs use preceptor-based systems, but few have consistently invested in the development and support of those preceptors. To be effective, preceptors require an educational foundation, ongoing support, and time to precept. A commitment to this time for teaching helps develop both preceptor and novice.

Our project identified two target audiences that require intensive education and support. First, the preceptor's teaching, mentoring, and competency assessment skills must be developed. A foundation must be laid with comprehensive, theory-based education related to interpersonal communication, roles/responsibilities, principles of teaching/learning, assessment, planning, and feedback skills. Once this foundation is laid, the preceptor's effectiveness should be evaluated on an ongoing basis in a system that focuses on performance development for both preceptors and novices. This process ensures the necessary structure for skills development and competency assessment that protects the safety of patients as well as the professional development of nurses.

The second target audience is the novice nurse. This nurse may be a new graduate, a reentry candidate, or a nurse transitioning into a new specialty area. Each of these novices needs advanced support, instruction, and precepting to develop the reflective learning, critical thinking, and specialty practice skills that are essential to safe, effective nursing care in multiple settings.

In summary, investment in these target groups has paid dividends for the state of Vermont. Dividends are in the form of recruitment, retention, and improved satisfaction for Vermont nurses.

7

Using Data to Influence Nursing Workforce Policy

*Eileen T. O'Grady, Geri Dickson,
Kathryn V. Hall, Marge Hegge,
Kim Welch Hoover, Ellen M. Lewis,
and Marcella M. McKay*

The trend toward evidenced-based policy formulation has increased the demand for research that provides clear, concise policy-relevant findings. To garner the power of existing workforce research (with gaps and all), nurses must link research findings to the health policy triad: access, quality, and cost. That is, each policy recommendation based on nursing workforce research must be associated with at least one of the three policy catalysts, increased quality and access to care and decreased health care costs (Wakefield, 2003).

Data on the nursing workforce alone are not enough to influence the policy-making process. Interpreting nursing workforce data and crafting thoughtful policy solutions serve the public by contributing to improved problem identification and specified solutions. Pertinent research findings can influence the agenda and bring forward health policy issues that have languished at the bottom of the policy agenda for years. A prerequisite for evidence-based policy formulation is effective communication of credible and current information to policy makers.

Governmental sources of data are the most credible because they are derived from a neutral source. These data sources should be used and linked to nursing research data at every opportunity. Once a policy maker perceives that the data are not credible, the opportunity to influence policy is lost. Demographic research, for example, continues to produce a large body of scientific knowledge that addresses critical issues faced by policy makers; however, the degree to which such research is translated into policy is highly dependent on how the findings are linked to policy recommendations and how those recommendations are communicated. This chapter describes the context for developing and using the evidence base for policy formulation, especially with regard to nursing workforce issues. Specific examples from states illustrate how data have been used recently to influence nursing workforce policy—both successfully and, at least in the case of California, unsuccessfully despite the eloquent collection, analysis, and dissemination of workforce data.

LINKING DATA TO POLICY

The defining purpose of health policy, as far as the government is concerned, is to support the citizenry in their quest for health. Most U.S. health policy problems that policy makers perceive as unimportant, conflict laden, or unsolvable never get addressed (Longest, 2002). Policy is often crafted on the basis of deeply held perceptions that may have been shaped by personal experience, anecdotes, actual facts, or from biased information supplied by interest groups.

In the past, relating research to policy was a linear process. The focus was on overcoming the distance between "knowledge-producers" (researchers) and "knowledge-consumers" (policy makers). The assumption was that research is directly useful to policies and that therefore the solution lies in strengthening the flow of knowledge from researchers so that it reaches policy makers intact. It is now understood, however, that the links between data driven research and policy making are not direct, and usually no single piece of data is likely to influence a policy change directly. Rather, data often influence policy through the cumulative weight of information, which leads to a gradual change in the thinking of policy makers. The exchange of information between researchers and policy makers is highly dynamic. Research introduces new concepts and therefore incrementally alters the language used in policy circles. Glimpses of new ideas and approaches may slightly alter the perception and understanding of policy makers. Therefore, even though research findings are not directly employed in a specific policy, they still—overall—exert a relatively powerful influence over the terms used and the way issues are framed and understood. Weiss (1977) called this the "enlightenment function" of research. She also described a visual image, "percolation," which refers to the way in which research findings and concepts circulate and gradually infiltrate policy discourse.

Types of Research

Research used for policy development comes in three forms. Research as data and findings is often presented as statistics or academic reports. Policy makers will only use this information if it addresses a specific identified problem answered by the statistics, supports a policy change favored by the policy maker, or highlights an immediate acute problem. Research as ideas and criticism involves the gradual flow of information and ideas through researchers and policy makers. Issues arising from the research gradually permeate the policy process through various channels, and it is difficult to identify the specific piece of research that leads to a policy change. Briefs and arguments for action are used when the researcher adopts the role of advocate. This type of research provides the policy maker with a set of alternatives to current problems. Briefs and arguments for action are the method the nursing community should employ as it distills research into specific policy recommendations. Policy makers will only seek research findings when they have a specific question. Consequently, the most critical strategy in linking research to policy is to involve policy makers at each stage of the research process. This collaboration fosters ownership of the research and ensures that the research is policy relevant (Porter & Prysor-Jones, 1997).

EXEMPLAR #1—BENCHMARKING IN THE STATE OF KENTUCKY

Benchmarking data are extremely useful tools to depict one's position with respect to larger and broader entities. Benchmarking—comparing local data to national data—is critical for effectively and proactively managing sound nursing workforce development. Benchmarking links the health care needs of the state population (or region) to those of the national population and then links both to nursing workforce data. Increasingly, a range of population-specific characteristics such as increased consumer access to information, prevalence of chronic illness, geographic population shifts, and changes in demographic, racial, and ethnic composition will collectively alter demands on the nursing workforce. For example, by the year 2050, the population of racial and ethnic minorities in the United States is expected to grow to almost 50% (U.S. Bureau of Labor Statistics, 2002). Changes in demographic characteristics coupled with disparate geographic distributions of nurses point to a demand for nurses in every sector of the delivery system. The link between the census data and characteristics of a strong nursing workforce may not be readily evident to a policy maker who is concerned about a broad range of public issues.

Integrating population demographic data, health care needs of the citizenry, and nurse resources at the state level is a necessary strategy in the quest to influence meaningful nursing workforce planning and policy (Malloch, Davenport, & Hatler, 2003). The following benchmark examples using data derived from nurse researchers in Kentucky compared those data to national data. The examples highlight evidenced-based policy recommendations incorporating access, cost, and quality concerns. (See Table 7.1.) The examples include evidenced-based policy recommendations that could be made.

Benchmarking and Policy Recommendations

Examples

Leading Cause of Death. In Kentucky, cardiovascular (CV) disease is the leading cause of death, indicating a high incidence of preventable disease. Patients with CV disease require a multipronged approach, beginning with prevention through rehabilitation and long-term care. Often, when the disease presents itself at midlife, intense nursing care is initially required followed by chronic nursing care. More nurses will be needed to improve the acute management as well as chronic care of patients with CV diseases. In addition, the CV disease rate requires a concerted public education campaign to reduce the incidence of the disease. Placing more nurses in the workplace, schools, and communities is an important strategy to reduce the burden of CV diseases on the community. The policy recommendation follows:

- Funding is needed for scholarships for basic nursing education and fast-track second-degree programs to increase the number of RNs in the state.
- Enhanced funding is needed to develop chronic illness care. More public health, acute care rehabilitation, and long-term care nurses will be required to combat the high rates of CV disease in the state.

TABLE 7.1   Benchmarking in Kentucky

Variable	National (Based on 2000 data)	Kentucky
3 Leading Causes of Death	1. Cardiovascular disease 2. All cancers 3. Stroke	1. Cardiovascular diseases 2. All Cancers 3. Stroke
Population over age 85	241/100,000	270/100,000
Average RN age	44.3 years	43.6 years
Diploma prepared RNs	23%	13%
Ethnic minority population	31%	8%
Ethnic minority nurses	13.3 %	3.3%

Sources: U.S. Department of Health and Human Services, 2004. Malloch, Davonport, & Hatler, 2003. U.S. Department of Health and Human Services, 2002.

Growing Elderly Population. The unprecedented growth in the number of older adults living in Kentucky relates directly to the need for more nurses. According to a 2004 Centers for Disease Control and Prevention (CDC) report, by age 80, up to 47% of the population will have one or more limitations that render them unable to live independently (U.S. Department of Health and Human Services, Centers for Disease Control and Prevention, 2004). Nursing services for all types of nurses, especially nurses who work with the geriatric population, will be required. Kentucky's population of those over 85 is growing at a faster rate than the national average. This population's shift will require more nurses in the delivery sectors that care for this population, such as home care and long-term care. The geriatric population requires nurses with expertise to manage the frail elderly with multiple acute and chronic health problems. Nurses with geriatric expertise enhance quality of care by preventing unnecessary hospitalizations and focusing on functional enhancement. The policy recommendation follows:

- Fund nursing scholarships for entering BSN students as well as gerontological nurse practitioners to educate more nurses specializing in gerontology.
- Convene a task force at the State Office on Aging to look at innovative strategies for enhancing the gerontological nursing workforce.

The Aging Nursing Workforce. The average age of Kentucky's nursing workforce is 43.6 years, only 7 months younger than the national average of nurses. Due to the physical demands of nursing, most nurses do not wait until 65 to retire, and therefore this state will be facing an acute shortage as these nurses retire within 10 years. High turnover rates are exceedingly costly to nursing employers. Implementing effective retention strategies reduces costs and increases quality of care. The state has a lower percentage of diploma-prepared RNs compared to the national average. However, as nursing becomes more complex, nurses require strong critical analytic and problem-solving skills, which are developed at the BSN and advanced practice nursing (APN) level. There is consensus that the diploma is not the appropriate level of RN preparation.[*] The policy recommendation follows:

- Provide funding to explore strategies that lessen the physical demands of nursing so that nurses are able to participate in the workforce longer.
- Redirect state and federal monies that now fund diploma nursing programs to fund baccalaureate nursing degree or advanced practice nursing programs.

Ethnic and Cultural Diversity. Kentucky has an 8% ethnic minority population and a 3.3% RN ethnic minority population (Malloch, Davenport, & Hatler, 2003). It is well known that patients whose caregivers are culturally matched have better overall health outcomes and higher quality of care. The policy recommendation follows:

---

[*]In response to shifting nursing workforce demands, the Division of Nursing's National Advisory Council on Nursing Education and Practice (NACNEP) called for a workforce with the capacity to adapt to change and use communication, critical-thinking, problem-solving and analysis skills that incorporate knowledge from the basic, behavioral, social, and management sciences. To address the demand for enhanced skills, the NACNEP recommended restructuring the nursing workforce by 2010 to achieve a goal in which two-thirds of the nursing workforce would hold a baccalaureate or higher education degree.

- Provide funding for cultural competency programs to enhance the skills and education of nurses already in practice.
- Fund programs with proven effectiveness to recruit ethnic and racial minorities into nursing so that the state population is culturally matched with the RN workforce.

Turning Recommendations into Policy

The examples provide powerful information to policy makers and help to delineate funding priorities. The data also set the legislative priorities for state and national nursing organizations that are developing the sophistication, analytic ability, and political competence to translate these benchmarks into effective nursing workforce policy. Using the U.S. Census as the source of data, rather than nursing-derived data, adds credibility to the policy argument and provides national perspective. Adding poignant stories or experiences that underscore these data will also add considerable strength to the workforce policy recommendations.

Funding Comparisons

Another form of benchmarking includes comparing federal funding levels for nursing with that for other disciplines. This technique clarifies issues for policy makers and helps define inequities. Medicare is the largest single source of federal support for nursing education. Unlike graduate medical education, Medicare supports primarily diploma education in nursing. Graduate nursing education, including the preparation of advanced practice nurses, does not generally qualify for graduate medical education funding. Curiously, while there is broad consensus that more BSN nurses are needed, the majority of Medicare nursing education funding goes to hospitals affiliated with diploma nurse training programs. In 2003, Medicare supported the costs of training resident physicians with direct and indirect Graduate Medical Education funds amounting to $7.1 billion per year. Compare that to the $200 million that Medicare funneled to nursing education, mostly to several northeastern states operating hospital diploma programs (Wandishin, J., personal communication, February 2004). This is an order of magnitude that is staggering, and many policy makers are unaware of how much Medicare supports physician education. As the care delivery system evolves, nursing could make a strong policy recommendation that Medicare reimbursement for nursing education must be retargeted to fund the training of graduate health care providers other than physicians who care for the Medicare population in hospitals (Aiken & Gwyther, 1995).

Scenario Development

Scenario development is another technique that forecasts a plausible, data-informed story about the future. This technique is especially amenable to situations that include baseline data with future uncertainties and imponderables. The essence of scenario development is to outline several alternative future scenarios so that a full range of possibilities is reflected. The scenario that appears to be the most probable future can form the basis of health policy solutions.

Political Competence

The ability to analyze and influence health policy effectively is termed *political competence*. Effective health policy making requires a thorough understanding of the health policy making process, which is a decision-making process. Decision making by policy makers is incremental, and they prefer to consider a relatively few alternatives that bring about marginal change on existing policies. By understanding the incremental policy making process and the views of the stakeholders, politically competent people know the timing and strategy at which they can be involved in the process. Understanding the process and the participants allows these individuals to engage effectively in the policy making process. Politically competent people can be involved in agenda setting, policy refinement, and rule making by providing relevant data, offering solutions to problems, drafting legislation, and providing testimony. Diffusing strategically important information on the nursing workforce and linking it to the broader current policy contexts, such as the focus on health care quality, is how the politically competent effectively influence policy makers. Once a thorough understanding of the health policy maker's process is known and the nursing workforce data have been analyzed, it is time to engage the policy maker. Some specific recommendations are summarized below and were actualized in the Colleagues in Caring stories that follow.

- *Package and interpret the data.* When presenting data to policy makers, make several simply worded policy recommendations. It is important to distill academic reports and peer-reviewed journal articles into bulleted, one-page summaries that include policy recommendations.
- *Take advantage of lead time.* The ability to develop effective responses—whether new policies or modifications—is greatly enhanced by lead time. This skill requires nurse leaders to

anticipate policy changes months ahead of when they actually occur, making it possible to have more thoughtful, evidenced-based, and appropriate policy recommendations.

- *Include policy makers in the nursing workforce research process.* Nursing leaders are responsible for supplying policy makers with data. This responsibility includes seeking the advice of the policy maker before, during, and after the data are collected and analyzed, thus raising the chance that the research will be policy relevant. Know what legislators are interested in and work effectively with their staff.
- *Whenever possible, use government sources to strengthen policy recommendations.* Using neutral, authoritative sources such as the reports from the Department of Health and Human Services, the Institute of Medicine, the Bureau of the Census, and the Bureau of Labor Statistics adds merit and power to support meaningful nursing workforce planning and can reframe policy issues.
- *Remove emotional arguments, and base policy recommendations on data.* At all costs, avoid being a shrill (overly strident, self-serving). Avoid appearing self-serving by connecting all policy recommendations to the policy triad of increased access and quality or decreased costs.
- *Make the data come alive.* Connect the data findings to the policy maker's community through poignant stories. Poignant stories differ from emotional arguments in that stories amplify the impact of a health care problem on real people and communities. This humanizing approach brings more meaning to the data and creates interest in policy recommendations.
- *Use data in letters to the editors of local newspapers.* Policy makers at all levels of government read their local newspapers to keep abreast of constituent issues. This strategy has a twofold impact by making both the public and the policy makers increasingly aware of health care problems and possible solutions.
- *Integrity is currency in the health policy-making process.* If you are unsure of an answer to a question from a policy maker, say so and follow up later with the referenced answer.

Future Challenges

Using data to inform nursing workforce policy is challenging. Currently, there are wide gaps in national nursing workforce data and a lack of generalizable findings that link population outcomes with specific nursing care. The National Sample Survey of Registered Nurses (NSSRN), an important source of data on the RN workforce, could be strengthened in a number of ways to better inform policy makers. Nursing leaders are challenged to believe they can make a difference and effectively influence sound workforce policies. Nursing's voice is sorely needed and belongs in the public policy discourse, as evidenced by the Colleagues in Caring successes. Nurses are challenged to get a seat at the policy-making table, come prepared with credible data, translate those data into policy recommendations, and conduct themselves in a manner that gets them invited back to the table.

EXEMPLAR #2—POLITICAL REALITIES OF POLICY CHANGE: THE SOUTH DAKOTA EXPERIENCE

Nursing workforce planning is only effective if it influences public policy to improve supply and demand of nurses. The challenges of translating data into political influence are daunting. Once political debates reach the public, those challenges take on unpredictable dimensions that are impossible to control. To prevail, a nursing workforce center needs the following tools: powerful partners, credible data, impeccable timing, passionate stories, eye-catching fact sheets, rational responses to opposition, and follow-through strategies.

The South Dakota Nursing Workforce Center, which began as a Robert Wood Johnson Foundation Colleagues in Caring project, was successful in passing three critical bills through the conservative South Dakota legislature in the 2002 economically depressed session. One bill increased nurse relicensure fees to fund a permanent nursing workforce center. A second bill expanded enrollment in the state public associate degree and baccalaureate nursing programs, whereas a third bill provided funds to reward nurses who practiced for two years in South Dakota facilities following graduation. Lessons learned during the successful campaign to pass these bills are shared below.

Components of a Successful Political Campaign

Powerful Partners

To advocate for passage of these bills, we created the South Dakota Consortium, which involved collaboration of nursing education, practice, and regulation. Representation from all 12 nursing programs (public, and private for associate's through master's degrees) was ensured in every working group. The three major health systems were invited to send practicing nurses to all meetings, and they consistently did so. Small rural facilities were also represented. Also invited were major practice settings, including long-term care, clinic, home health/hospice, mental health, public health, and school health. The state's nursing organizations were all represented at the table, from the licensed practical nurse (LPN) association through advanced practice nurse (APN) associations like the nurse anesthetists. In addition, the state board of nursing was an active partner in all meetings, as were the state regulatory agencies of the departments of health, labor, mental health, and education. Convening all these partners created a scheduling challenge with a shifting group of attendees. Efforts were made to keep all partners informed and involved through minutes, draft documents, and a Web-site.

Three consumer members were invited to join the consortium, one from the state disabilities coalition, one from the American Association of Retired Persons, and the other from the state chapter of the National Association for the Mentally Ill. They actively participated in discussions by adding the client and family perspectives on health issues and nursing practice.

Interdisciplinary colleagues were also important partners. Insurance executives, physicians, administrators, pharmacists, and social workers added valuable perspectives to the dialogue. In South Dakota, the major professional organizations for these groups were asked to send representatives, who attended sporadically depending on agenda items in which they had an interest. Occasionally, they provided written feedback on drafts.

Two legislators, one Republican and one Democrat, were named to the consortium, one from the house and the other from the senate. They provided valuable insights into legislative processes, timing, and coalition building. The governor, secretary of health, and Department of Labor officials were critical advocates for nursing legislation. Their influence, credibility, and networks were instrumental in building public support for the nursing bills. All reports were shared with the U.S. senators and representatives, who used data in legislative efforts to pass the Nurse Reinvestment Act at the federal level.

Credible Data

The quest for sound data begins with the right questions—those partners really care about. Once the partners determine the most important questions, data systems and strategies can be designed to find answers. Tools should be feasible, brief, and pertinent. The methodology should begin with what data already exits. Comparison points should be used to trend data over time. Whenever data can be verified by another agency, the data become more robust politically, avoiding the perception that nurses are spinning the data to build a case for more funds for themselves.

Most legislators reject national data extracted to the state. They prefer to have local and statewide data collected by their own citizens. Whenever information can be tailored for individual counties or regions, it will catch the attention of legislators from those areas.

The importance of one official version of the data cannot be underestimated. Select a freeze date and capture the data that day. Build all material from this official version to avoid conflicting data from a rolling data set.

Impeccable Timing

Start the political process early to build momentum, at least two years before anticipated action. Legislator members advised the consortium about competing budget items and other dominant issues and key leadership priorities, so that the nursing bills fit into a larger context of health care, insurance, and rural infrastructure reform. National and state media coverage of the growing nursing shortage built public awareness of workforce issues, and therefore legislators and their constituents were primed for action on nursing. Unity among the nursing community is crucial. Many meetings and lots of discussion are needed to achieve this consensus. Nothing kills a legislative effort quicker than public infighting among nurses.

Passionate Stories

Nothing propels political action better than personal testimony. During the hearings, the following stories influenced votes:

- A nurse testified that she would not have gone to nursing school without significant financial aid to support her family while she was enrolled full time in class and clinical rotations.
- A former nurse relayed her disappointment that she was compelled to leave the field due to continual expectations to work overtime because of persistent nursing shortages. The pressure threatened to dissolve her marriage, and she made the hard choice to leave nursing due to unrealistic workplace demands.
- A rural hospital administrator shared his fear that the two core RNs staffing his facility were nearing retirement age with

no replacements in sight, jeopardizing the viability of the only
health center in the county.
- An urban director of nursing reported that experienced RNs
were being recruited out of state in alarming numbers by
employers offering large bonuses and significantly higher
salaries.

Eye-Catching Fact Sheets

One-page summaries of the most pertinent arguments are essential. They should be colorful, graphic, and bumper-sticker simple.
They should contain sound bites that can convey the central messages, such as the following:

> Quality care depends on experienced RNs. There will not be
> enough to staff our facilities unless we act now. What can be done?
> Expand nursing program enrollments, reward nurses who practice
> two years in the state, establish a nursing workforce center.

A Web-site URL should be clearly visible for more information.

Rational Responses to Opposition

In any political campaign, opponents will challenge data, counter
arguments, or debate the merits of the proposal. Their motivation is
usually economic. Some are self-appointed guard dogs at the door of
the state treasury. Others are promoting their own proposals competing for the same funds. Still others believe their constituents who
claim there is no nursing shortage in their hospital. Whatever the
source of opposition, a rational response is indicated. Be respectful of
adversaries while challenging them with facts, figures, and data. Build
deep enough campaign strategies so that several legislators are prepared to counter arguments to demonstrate a broad base of support.

Follow-Through Strategies

Celebrate achievements, thank those who carried the momentum, and
evaluate the process. Those who invested in nursing have a right to
know what a difference they made. Plans should be made to track
nursing workforce changes to show a positive impact.

The ongoing analysis of turnover rates, vacancies, nurse retention,
NCLEX (the licensing examinations for registered nurses and practical nurses) pass rates, and job placement of new graduates should
all reflect the pivotal legislative decision to invest in nursing. This
feedback will enhance the credibility of the nursing workforce center
and those who believed in it. Such reports will go a long way in
preparation for subsequent legislative issues.

Top 10 Tips for Influencing Public Policy

1. Get control of your own data with a freeze date and one official version.
2. Translate it into bumper-sticker-simple sound bites.
3. Link to official government agencies for depth and credibility.
4. Be shameless in contacting officials for support early and often.
5. Anticipate opposition and counter with air-tight arguments.
6. Do whatever it takes to avoid nurses fighting nurses in public.
7. Tell stories that pull at the heartstrings.
8. Start early and pepper the state with media coverage of nursing issues.
9. Persist no matter how impossible it seems.
10. Follow through with celebration and thanks.

Political processes inspire the overachiever in all of us. They build confidence and they convince us we can do the impossible if we stick together and persevere.

EXEMPLAR #3—CALIFORNIA MINUS THE GOLD: NURSING WORKFORCE LEGISLATION

The California Strategic Planning Committee for Nursing (CSPCN) was formed in 1992 as an unincorporated consortium. Its purpose was to develop reliable nursing workforce data for public policy and resource allocation decisions to meet California's need for nurses. This section focuses on the legislative journey of CSPCN as it worked to accomplish its goals over the past decade.

State of the State—Historical View

At the time CSPCN was initiated, California and the health care delivery system were in crisis. The state was suffering through a severe financial budget crisis. The defense industry was declining and military bases were closing because the cold war, for the most part, had ended. The Los Angeles area was recovering from the Northridge Earthquake, and Laguna Beach was rebuilding after a horrific fire and devastation in that region of southern California. If that were not enough, the health care delivery system and reimbursement for care were being reinvented on a daily basis. At least that is how patients, providers, and payers perceived the changes in the

health care system. Every day newspapers reported that professional nurses were being laid off from their positions as hospitals
downsized, reorganized, merged, or were bought by corporations.

In the late 1990s, the state began to turn around with the Silicon
Valley "dot.com" explosion. This lasted for several years, and nursing leaders in the state hoped health care would reap benefits from all
the revenue being generated by the state due to a healthy economy.
However, the energy crisis occurred and rolling blackouts were frequent and recurring nightmares. To make matters worse, the nation
experienced 9/11, the Enron scandal, and the bubble-burst of the
dot.com era. California, which had the eighth largest economy in
the world, found itself back in a severe deficit situation because the
surplus of revenue generated during the dot.com era had to be used
to fund costly energy contracts that were signed by Governor Davis
(D) to help alleviate the energy crisis. Gray Davis was recalled, and
the new Governor, Arnold Schwartzenegger, is charged with creating
financial solvency once again.

Between 1994 and 2002, a turbulent and glorious economic time
in California, CSPCN started establishing a database to describe the
supply and demand for nurses in California. In 1989, the California legislature had appointed the RN Special Advisory Committee to study
issues confronting the profession and to make recommendations
for change. This committee submitted its report to the legislature in
1990, which included 12 recommendations. The report was accepted
by the legislature but was not funded; therefore, none of the recommendations was acted upon. Recommendation 5 of the report was to
establish a master plan for nursing manpower and education to
ensure an adequate supply of nurses. CSPCN took this recommendation and made it the driving force for its activity. CSPCN believed
from the beginning that California did not have adequate program
capacity to educate the numbers of nurses it would need to meet
the demand because there had been no permanent change in nursing education slots and no commitment for change in decades.

Data collected through the efforts of CSPCN (Sechrist, Lewis,
Rutledge, 1999) found that the proportion of RNs per 100,000 population was already among the lowest in the nation. The RN workforce
continued to age, and less than 10% of the workforce were under 30
years of age and 30% of the workforce were over 50 years of age. Of
RNs with active California RN licenses who were living in California,
85% worked full or part time, which is higher than the national average. California already relied on other states and countries for 50% of
its nursing workforce at a time when international and national
shortages were being reported. California's associate degree and

baccalaureate RN prelicensure programs were universally fully sub-scribed annually. An increasing shortage of faculty further contributed to the problem. Employers continued to report the need for additional BSN- and graduate-degree-prepared nurses. Approximately 70% of RNs educated in California graduated from associate degree pro-grams. On average, only 20% of associate degree nurses continued their education for a baccalaureate or higher degree in nursing (16% in 1997) or another field. California's ethnic/racial diversity was not reflected in the current RN nursing workforce. However, the ethnic/racial background of students enrolled in prelicensure pro-grams was more closely aligned with the ethnic/racial background of the population. There was one notable exception: The propor-tion of Hispanic/Latino students lagged behind the proportion of Hispanics/Latinos in the population.

In 1998, the Department of Labor (U.S. Bureau of Labor Statistics, 1998) and the California Employment Development Department (State of California, Employment Development Department, Labor Market Information, 1998) listed RNs and licensed vocational nurses (LVNs) among occupations with the largest expected growth by 2006. The California Employment Development Department projected an absolute growth of 39,470 RN and 19,970 LVN jobs for the period 1996–2006. This may be an extremely conservative esti-mate because California's population is expected to increase by over 17 million individuals by 2025 with half of the increase coming from foreign migration. CSPCN survey findings conducted in 1996, 1999, and 2002 all predicted current and future shortages in the workforce as well as faculty shortages. All reports that were gener-ated by these surveys were widely disseminated through statewide summits, regional and national meetings, testimony before the Institute of Medicine, the California legislature, and multiple peer-reviewed publications. CSPCN's efforts to influence policy related to workforce planning for California are detailed below.

Public Policy Initiatives

In 1998, a bill was introduced to appropriate $145,000 from the Board of Registered Nursing Fund to that board to conduct an assess-ment of the demographics of the nursing workforce in California in relation to the population of the state and to make recommenda-tions to the legislature regarding nurse education and training pro-grams in the state (California State University, 1998; Keating & Sechrist, 2001). This bill would have provided financial support for CSPCNs workforce initiative and a home for CSPCN in one of the state government departments or offices. Research findings supported the bill, and it passed almost unanimously but was then vetoed by the governor Wilson.

Another bill in 1999 formed the Scott Commission and required that the chancellors of the community colleges, the chancellor of California State University, the president of the University of California, and the president of the Association of Independent Colleges and Universities jointly issue a report to the governor and the legislature with respect to a recommended plan, alternative strategies, and a budget for significantly increasing the number of students graduating from nursing programs in the state and for providing specialty training to licensed nurses in prescribed areas of specialization. CSPCN provided the data that were used to support the need for this bill. This bill was passed by the legislature and signed into law by Governor Davis. Conventional wisdom exists that he signed the bill in error because he thought it was a nurse-staffing bill. CSPCN's chair, project investigator, and project director served as 3 of the 20 members of the commission. CSPCN's survey data were incorporated into the report. Recommendations of the Scott Commission included increased funding for state-supported programs, increased financial aid for students, integration of CSPCN into the Board of Registered Nursing, and increased recruitment efforts. The commission completed its work in a timely manner; however, the chancellors delayed submitting the report for over three months. Eventually $15 million were placed into the state budget to support recommendations during revisions of the Budget process. Unfortunately, owing to pressure from the chancellors, the governor line-item vetoed the funds. A separate line item designated a small amount for one-time technical support for "expensive programs," i.e., computer science, engineering, and nursing, but was not to be used to increase enrollments in any of these programs. Once again, great work and great recommendations were left unfunded.

In October 1999, the governor signed into law a bill that required the department of health services to set ratios for RN staffing in the state of California. This was the first such legislation in the nation. These ratios were first envisioned and introduced into legislature in 1992 but took seven years to get to the governor's desk for signature. The impact of this legislation on the demand for nurses was predicted to be significant, and the data continued to indicate the same issues that plagued supply; i.e., insufficient space in California nursing programs and immigration from other states and foreign countries.

Efforts continued, however, in the state legislature to increase the supply of nurses in the state. In 2000, an assemblyman introduced a bill to create a demonstration project partnering industry and education in Orange County, California. The bill would have provided $1.7 million to be matched by hospitals to increase the number of RN graduates. No action was taken on this bill after the second reading. In 2001, another bill was introduced in an effort to direct educational systems to standardize all nursing program prerequisites statewide. This work was to be in conjunction with the statewide Intersegmental Major Preparation Articulated Curriculum project. This bill was carried over to the next legislative session and, to date, has not been addressed. Clearly external events, i.e. the energy crisis, 9/11 and Enron turned the focus away from the nursing shortage issues, but the much delayed and publicized staffing ratio legislation brought the shortage issues to public attention.

In 2001, a bill was introduced in the legislature and was approved. This legislation (Work Force Training Act) made $1 million available to community colleges to fund specialty training of RNs, and the senate added $4 million in appropriations for additional community college nursing programs. This was the first real money to be added to fund nursing education in over a decade. Legislators up for reelection in 2002 continued to court the nursing unions and other nursing and health groups hoping for their support and vote. Several nursing shortage legislative hearings were held during this same period, but unfortunately, little or nothing happened.

Then on January 23, 2002, Governor Davis announced the Nurse Workforce Initiative (NWI) to address California's growing nursing shortage. NWI promised $60 million over three years in support of nursing education. Included in this $60 million allocation were $8 million that already had been given to the Central Valley Region of California by a private grantor. NWI also incorporated both short-term and long-term measures to build and sustain a culturally diverse nursing workforce to meet California's health care needs. It proposed a speedier process for RN license applications (E-Applications) and extended the duration of temporary licenses from 18 months to 2 years. To the extent possible, the NWI would rely on funding from the Federal Workforce Investment Act (WIA). Further, NWI would use funds from the Employment Training Panel to support those activities that complement the training activities supported by WIA. Also, the governor aimed to engage private foundations in funding certain aspects of NWI. To date, approximately $26 million of the $60 million have been allocated to collaborative ventures between WIA and educational institutions.

With the removal of Governor Davis from office and the present state budget deficit, the NWI is in limbo with little hope that it will be resurrected.

In 2002, CSPCN and its activities of data collection and strategic planning for nursing education in California were subsumed into activities of the board of registered nursing (BRN). The newly appointed BRN nursing workforce and educational advisory committees will continue to collect and report supply and demand data as well as make recommendations related to nursing education and curriculum.

So Where's the Gold?

California faces significant challenges to provide an adequately prepared nursing workforce for the future. CSPCN, other nursing stakeholders, and policy makers have advocated, introduced, and sometimes been successful in creating legislative redress for the nursing shortage in California. The "gold," however, remains elusive. However, it is clear that if no new money is available to address the lack of supply of nurses in California, policy makers will need to make tough decisions about resource allocation for health care. If funds are not provided for nursing education, California will face a health care crisis that will threaten the lives of its people. To avoid this crisis, existing programs will need to be expanded and new programs established. In addition, action must be taken to increase the number of faculty qualified to teach in the new and expanded programs. In the meantime, balancing nurse supply with demand and complying with ratios is extremely challenging for health care provider organizations and nurse leaders.

EXEMPLAR #4—CREATION OF THE MARYLAND STATEWIDE COMMISSION ON THE CRISIS IN NURSING

The most recent nursing shortage in Maryland began between 1997 and 1999. In 1999 more than 2,300 nurses with active licenses failed to renew those licenses to practice nursing in the state (Maryland Commission on the Crisis in Nursing, 2001). Further, in 1997, data from the Maryland Board of Nursing revealed a leveling off in the supply of nurses. Moreover, enrollments in nursing education programs were dropping, and most of the community college nursing programs were below capacity. The Maryland Colleagues in Caring (MCIC) project found, through its collection of demand data, that acute care settings across the state were experiencing inadequate nursing staff in the operating rooms, the emergency rooms, and intensive care units. A few general medical/surgical units were also beginning to experience a shortage of nursing staff.

Because of the growing concern that more nurses would soon retire from the profession than would enter, some key interest groups came together to draft legislation to establish the Statewide Commission on the Crisis in Nursing. These interest groups believed that creating the commission would increase the policy makers' and public's awareness of the growing shortage of nurses. The Maryland Board of Nursing, the Maryland Hospital Association, and the Maryland Colleagues in Caring were among the leaders in this effort. Bills were introduced in the 2000 Maryland Legislative Session (Senate Bill 311 and House Bill 363) that created a 45-member commission representing not only the nursing community but also the Maryland Higher Education Commission, the broader health care community, and the public. The legislation created the commission for a period of five years to allow for better development and evaluation of strategies to address this potential health care crisis.

As set forth by the legislation, the commission's functions were to do the following:

- Convene a summit to respond to the nursing shortage.
- Determine the current extent and long-term implications of the growing nursing shortage.
- Evaluate mechanisms currently available in the state and elsewhere that are intended to enhance education, recruitment, and retention of nurses in the workplace and to improve quality of care.
- Assess the impact of the shortage on access to and the delivery of quality patient care.
- Develop recommendations and facilitate the implementation of strategies to reverse the growing shortage, including (1) determining what changes are needed in existing scholarship programs and (2) funding mechanisms to better reflect and accommodate the changing health care delivery environment and to improve the quality of care to meet the needs of patients.
- Facilitate career advancement within nursing.
- Accurately identify specific shortage areas in a timely manner.

- Attract middle and high school students into nursing as a career.
- Project a more positive and professional image of nursing and serve as an advisor to public and private entities to facilitate implementation of the recommendations of the commission.

In addition, the legislation called for the establishment of sub-committees on recruitment, retention, and education. A fourth sub-committee was added that would focus on workplace issues.

Work in many of these focus areas was also the focus of MCIC, and that work was made available to the Statewide Commission on the Crisis in Nursing. Many of the commissioners were also active par-ticipants in the MCIC project, and collectively the two groups had the unified mission of working to reverse the growing workforce shortage in the state. The project director for the MCIC project sat on the statewide commission as a vice-chair. The establishment of the commission elevated the awareness of nursing workforce issues in the minds of the members of the Maryland General Assembly. The commission met for the first time on August 30, 2000.

Data on both nursing supply and demand formed the basis for the beginning work for the commission. Recognized nationally for its work, the Maryland Board of Nursing maintains a thorough data-base on its licensees. Nursing licensure data were collected annually and captured not only the demographics of nurses in the state but also employment trends. The data clearly demonstrated that the largest cohort of practicing nurses was 38–47 years of age. Because the cohorts of younger nurses contained fewer numbers, the data indi-cated that there would be an even larger shortage once the baby boomers began to retire. The data also showed that the overall nursing workforce was not growing. The MCIC demand data indi-cated that most employers were projecting a greater need for nurses in both a three- and five-year projected time frames. Nurses themselves were reporting growing concerns about the work envi-ronment and increased employer demands. These concerns were confirmed by the more than 500 nurses who attended a statewide summit held in the first year of the commission's work.

In addition to examining the supply and demand data, the com-mission sought information on the status of nursing education. Some projects aimed at increasing enrollments in schools of nursing were already underway as part of the focus of the MCIC project, and the commission's interest in these initiatives lent support and emphasis to them. The education work group explored ways to increase scholarship money made available to qualified nursing school applicants, and legislation was introduced in the first year of the commission to expand state funding. Within three years, each of the 24 schools of nursing in the state were at or above capacity. Achieving capacity, of course, creates its own set of problems with availability of nursing faculty, clinical practice settings, and actual space for classes at the schools.

In addition to examining educational issues, the commission assessed concerns regarding retention of qualified nursing staff. The commission brokered a benefits and compensation study to begin to address some of those concerns across employment settings.

The commission continues its work in the state, and although enrollments and graduations of nursing students have improved, they are not keeping pace with the drain of nurses leaving the workforce. Capacity in the schools and availability of nursing faculty seem to be the areas of most concern at this time. The idea of forming an entity beyond the commission that would focus uniquely on nursing is once again being entertained.

Lessons Learned

The formation of a statewide commission was an excellent way to engage state lawmakers in the discussions around health care workforce needs and also to increase the awareness of the general population. For those areas that could best be dealt with legislatively, it afforded a great liaison to the Maryland General Assembly—for education and action.

The actual membership of the commission, however, was somewhat difficult because *every* nursing group and specialty wanted representation. Consequently, the commission became a group of nearly 50 people. The large size made development of strategic initiatives and action plans extremely difficult.

The leadership of the commission was equally problematic because of its size. Eight co-chairs provided oversight to the commission's work. Needless to say, we had a leadership challenge.

The law establishing the commission required that several members of the general assembly participate. Having policy makers at the table was very worthwhile because these individuals became the champions of nursing issues in the general assembly. They were instrumental in successfully proposing legislative initiatives from the commission, including a mandatory overtime bill and nursing scholarship bills.

Since the commission was a government entity, direct involvement of the private sector was limited. The commission worked to overcome this apparent obstacle by holding a summit and creating committees that brought in a large perspective of nursing workforce issues. As we look forward, we can use these lessons learned to form an entity that can bring the best of both the private and public sectors together to address the future health care workforce.

EXEMPLAR #5—HOW DATA INFLUENCE THE NURSING WORKFORCE AGENDA IN MISSISSIPPI

The Mississippi Office of Nursing Workforce (MONW) was formed in the mid-1990s as part of a statewide effort to prepare Mississippi nurses for managed care. This section describes how data became a leverage point for continuation of state funding for the MONW.

As MONW evolved, priorities shifted from its original vision, the reality of workforce redeployment issues, to workforce shortage issues that were quite evident in the national press. By 1999, workforce shortages were being reported across the United States and health care executives were focusing on national workforce demographics and projections of future shortages. The supply-and-demand data collection and reporting system developed by MONW was a valuable tool for Mississippi policy makers to determine regional and statewide nursing workforce trends and compare Mississippi to the country as a whole. The Colleagues in Caring (CIC) workforce data became a centerpiece for planning, implementing, and evaluating workforce initiatives statewide.

This national media blitz coincided with the end of the Robert Wood Johnson Foundation CIC stage II funding. The MONW advisory committee made the decision to continue the data collection and analysis as the highest priority of the office even if other initiatives had to be put on hold. In addition, the emphasis of MONW activities shifted to workforce issues, including recruitment and retention of both nursing students and faculty. MONW positioned itself to assume a primary role in public policy by ensuring a data system to support decision making based on unbiased information. At that time, Dr. Kim Hoover was brought in as executive director to ensure the continuation of the data system, and Judy Leavitt, a health policy expert, became the chair of the MONW advisory committee. The importance of strategic decision making at this point cannot be stressed enough. In fact, decisions involving the leadership of the office were crucial in ensuring its success.

The year 2000 was pivotal for MONW. Our budget was meager, and continuation of the office was questionable unless ongoing funding could be secured. The MONW advisory committee made a decision to pursue legislative funding, and Betty Dickson, executive director and lobbyist for the Mississippi Nursing Association (MNA), spearheaded the initiative, resulting in $100,000 in state funding. The MONW advisory committee developed a strategic plan with two fundamental goals: (1) to maintain a state-of-the-art data collection, analysis, and reporting system for the nursing workforce in Mississippi and (2) to seek grants and develop products/services in response to nursing workforce priorities to ensure the long-term financial viability of MONW. The year was spent searching for and hiring an executive director with the skills and characteristics needed to achieve self-sustainability and develop the role of the research/data specialist.

In 2001, Wanda Jones, MSN, RN, was hired as the executive director and Kim Hoover, PhD, RN, assumed the new role of director of research. Again, this was a deliberate decision to achieve specific goals for the organization. The executive director had experience with many different aspects of health care, hospital nursing, home health nursing, nursing education, and nursing administration. Consequently, she had a large network upon which to build relationships. This executive director had not previously been involved with MONW and therefore had no preconceived notion of where opportunities might present themselves. Her entrepreneurial spirit fostered creativity and allowed future planning to be unencumbered by past MONW experiences. In addition, the full development of an administrative role for data/research allowed concentration on the data system without distraction of responsibility for fund-raising and ongoing program development.

Betty Dickson, MNA executive director, continued to support the office through lobbying state legislators and coordinated a special legislative hearing focused on the nursing shortage at which MONW representatives provided expert testimony and data-driven presentations on supply, demand, and trends for the nursing workforce. The hearing was well attended by media representatives from newspapers and television. Health policy students at the baccalaureate and master's level attended sessions and talked with legislators. MONW increased the visibility of nursing workforce data and MONW priorities through presentations and handouts. The office provided leadership and exhibited the ability to be the credible source of reliable data on Mississippi nurses.

Concurrently, MONW's executive director explored other avenues of funding. Because health care entities and providers were major contributors to the Mississippi workforce and economy, the Mississippi Development Authority was targeted. This agency was the conduit in

Mississippi for federal workforce monies and recognized the expertise of MONW by agreeing to fund not only the data collection but two other major projects as well. Since that time, the legislature has continued to fund the data collection and other initiatives. Additional sources of income were sought through the development of revenue-generating products and services offered by MONW.

Relationship building that took almost five years to come to fruition has finally paid off. In the past two years, MONW has become the recognized source of credible nursing workforce data collection and analysis for the state of Mississippi. The data were gathered by individuals, groups, and agencies across the state and in other states for health care planning, grant writing, project development, and news articles. MONW has facilitated data collection and analysis for other groups and, in return, maintained a strong network of partners who shared data and supported MONW efforts.

MONW is involved in projects too numerous to detail here, but all rely heavily on successful data collection and influence. That success is based primarily on the following principles: diversity, leadership, timing, commitment, and relationship building (formal and informal). Diversity that extends beyond nursing stimulated creativity and original ideas and garnered financial support from nontraditional sources. Therefore, deliberate decisions regarding leadership are crucial and must involve a critical assessment of the skills needed to achieve the goals of the future, not just those of the moment. Maintaining current relationships while constantly cultivating new ones allowed opportunities for MONW to demonstrate its value to the overall health of the state and southeast region. All of those tactics were essential in establishing an unbiased, credible source of nursing data in the state. Using the data, seeking opportunities to share the data, and helping groups with common interests were just as important as building the database. More information on current and past MONW projects is available online (http://www.monw.org).

EXEMPLAR #6— DATA AS A DRIVER FOR CENTER CREATION IN NEW JERSEY

"Nurses are the backbone of the health care system," said Governor James E. McGreevey as he signed the bill to establish the New Jersey Collaborating Center for Nursing on December 12, 2002 (NJ chapter law 2002, c116). The road to the center began in 1995 with the Robert Wood Johnson Foundation Colleagues in Caring program, for which New Jersey was a grant recipient.

The Origin of the New Jersey Colleagues in Caring

New Jersey is a small, densely populated state, and meetings could be held in a central location. We started forming the New Jersey collaborative by bringing together stakeholder representatives of all sectors of nursing, including regulatory bodies and health policy makers. Commitment to the mission of CIC, creating change through the collaboration of nursing stakeholders, was the basis that brought us together and held us together during the first three years of the project, as well as in phase II (1999–2002), the next three years of the project. We found our experience similar to that of Flower (1995), who indicated that "if you bring together the appropriate people in constructive ways, with good information, they will create authentic visions and strategies for addressing the shared concern(s) of the participating organizations and community constituents" (p. 22).

The commitment and collaboration brought representatives from various aspects of nursing to the table in a state where the ramifications from the ANA 1965 Position Paper advocating two levels of nursing licensure are still felt keenly. As a means of organizing the work and defining a mission, vision, and purpose, the colleagues agreed to use the process of consensus. Coming to consensus was a process of dialogue and not of unanimity. Everyone had a voice; all were included because all members had made a commitment to dialogue and to stay at the table. Demand data and health policy work groups were established for developing a projection model to forecast the demand for nurses in New Jersey and for advocating the establishment of a legislatively mandated nursing workforce center.

Beginning the Journey to a Center

The data objective was to develop a dependable system for estimating the future demand for nurses in New Jersey. Demand, from an economic perspective, is the number of nurses that employers would be willing to hire, given their availability. Initially, we attempted to adapt the national Bureau of Health Professions nursing demand model to New Jersey. After many false starts, the bottom line was that it was not possible to adapt the national model for New Jersey. Therefore, we started again and developed a nursing demand forecasting model for New Jersey that would forecast the future demand for nurses and enable the schools of nursing to plan for a commensurate number of graduates to enter the workforce.

At the same time as the nursing demand model workgroup was creating the forecasting model, a health policy workgroup was developing a legislative network to seek legislation to create a state nursing workforce center. The workgroup developed three criteria that any center would need to meet: it must provide visibility for nursing, it must have credibility, and it must have neutrality (i.e., represent all walks of the nursing community). These three criteria also were steeped in the basic assumptions of CIC: commitment, collaboration, and consensus. Equally important was the need to communicate, communicate, communicate, which was done through quarterly newsletters, annual conferences, and, of course, the numerous work group meetings.

The members of the health policy workgroup were adamant that whatever the CIC became, it should provide a strong presence for nursing in the state. Leadership was seen as the key and it was clear, as Fagin (2000) suggested, that individual nurses want recognition, respect, and reward. Although nurses appreciate the intangible rewards of taking care of patients, what nurses want as professionals is "a place at the table of decision-making, and commensurate reward" (Abrams, 2002). Expanding and sustaining the work of the CIC project in the establishment of a center for nursing not only embodied the three criteria but fulfilled the mandate to be present at the table when decisions about nursing and health care are made.

As the nursing shortage heated up, we were able to develop four forecasts with the use of our demand model. The forecasts for 2006 included (a) the demand for the total number of RNs in the workforce, (b) the total number of LPNs in the workforce, (c) the full-time equivalent (FTE) positions for RNs in acute care only, and (4) FTEs for LPNs in acute care. At the same time, we had data on the supply of New Jersey working RNs and LPNs, as well as annual trend data for new graduates entering the workforce each year. The demand data and the supply data were then linked to estimate the gap between supply and demand for RNs and LPNs in the total workforce.

As we communicated with legislators, we began to educate them and lobbyists of the organizations of the collaborative, about the growing nursing shortage. Using the numbers from the demand-and-supply data, we were able to hypothesize that if (1) the New Jersey demand model was accurate in forecasting a demand for 11,000 new RN positions by 2006, (2) the number of New Jersey entry-level graduates continues to decrease, and (3) the rate of those leaving nursing continues at the usual rate of 3% per year, then New Jersey will be short nearly 14,000 RNs in 2006. This represents an RN vacancy rate of 18%. A 10% vacancy rate is considered a severe shortage. Continuing with the same assumptions, there would be 3,786 LPN positions unfilled by 2006 in the total LPN workforce, which is a 17% vacancy rate. These data were particularly useful in advancing the case to establish a center for nursing workforce development.

The Politics of Establishing a Center

After legislative networking and testimonies about the nursing shortage, legislation was introduced to establish the New Jersey Collaborating Center for Nursing in the 2001 session. The *"collaborating"* modifier was an important reminder of the legacy of the CIC project. The proposed legislation was patterned after that of the North Carolina Center for Nursing. The appropriation was $1.2 million, which included startup costs and first-year operating costs. The economy was good, and the chances looked good.

All the legislators were up for election in November of 2001. Before the elections, the governor and both houses were Republican; after the elections, there was a Democratic governor, a Democratic assembly, and a 50/50 split in the senate. The lame duck session was chaotic, and the center legislation died in committee in the 2001 session.

However, the bill was reintroduced in the 2002 senate session and referred to and, in March, released from the health committee. In June, just before the summer recess, the senate voted 40–0 to pass the bill. The bill was then introduced in the assembly and referred to the health committee, where an amendment was put forth. Both the bill and the amendment were released from the health committee and then passed by the assembly, However, it was returned to the senate for approval of the amendment, which was to increase the board to 17 members by adding a direct care RN to the board. Eventually, the bill made its way through the senate to the governor's desk. Governor James E. McGreevey signed the bill into law on December 12, 2002 (P.L. 2002, c116). There was just one small problem: the state now had a severe fiscal deficit and there was no appropriation attached to the bill.

Again, the Robert Wood Johnson Foundation rose to the challenge and funded the center through a two-year proposal that Dickson had written. Subsequently, the state did provide some funds that allowed us set up another year of funding. The center is located in Newark and is part of the College of Nursing of Rutgers, The State University of New Jersey. Current work and accomplishments of the center can be found on our Web-site (http:// www.njccn.org).

Lessons Learned

In looking back at the collaboration and activities that allowed us to become a nursing center, some things would be done differently today. The first lesson we learned was to check out your state's constitution to see how legislation is formed, the right language to use, and what restrictions might apply to you. For example, we used North Carolina as a template but later learned that the formation of the North Carolina Center could not occur in the same manner in New Jersey.

Another lesson learned was to consider carefully how members of the board of directors are to be selected or appointed. Since the legislation was written, we have found that different language would have made the appointment process easier. For example, just stating that the appointed members must be members of representative organizations, instead of being recommended by that particular organization, would make for a smoother appointment process.

All of our board members are public members. It would be helpful to have state commissioners, e.g., labor or education, or their designees, as representatives on the board. This would add a diversity of disciplines to the Board and allow for networking and sharing of knowledge among the state agencies.

Last, and most important, is the concept of collaboration. A solid base of collaboration, such as that provided by the Colleagues in Caring project, jump-starts the formation, visibility, credibility, and neutrality of a center. And certainly having adequate funding is crucial to the success of a center's endeavors. The right staff with the right talents also are critical to the center's success. Staff that are cross-trained, e.g., in research and administration, are extremely beneficial to the success of a center. Most important are people who are passionate about their responsibilities.

As more and more research evidence supports the importance of a link between nursing knowledge and practice and the safety and positive outcomes of patient care (e.g., Institute of Medicine, 2004), nurse leaders are poised to own nursing practice and demonstrate the difference that nursing can make. Fagin (1999) clearly emphasized this when she wrote, "The health of our health care system depends on nurses. To demean, diminish, or eliminate them puts the entire system in jeopardy" (p. F7).

8

Other Innovative Strategies for Nursing Workforce Development

Dennis R. Sherrod, James W. Bevill, and Barbara S. Mitchell

emand for registered nurses is skyrocketing. The U.S. Bureau of Labor Statistics (2004) recently announced that registered nurses rank number one in the nation's 10 growth occupations and are expected to demonstrate larger job growth than any other occupation in the United States between 2002 and 2012. Total job openings for registered nurses in that time are estimated to expand by more than 1.1 million. And this figure does not include needed replacements for retiring nurses. If necessity is the mother of invention, then this dramatic increase in nurse workforce demand surely requires innovative strategies and solutions.

The nurse workforce shortage is multifaceted, complex, interrelated, and unlike any we have experienced before. One solution will not resolve the shortage, and a myriad of creative recruitment and retention strategies will be required to ensure a qualified nurse workforce capable of meeting our population's evolving health care needs.

WORKPLACE RETENTION

One of the most important concepts in workforce development is retention. And although both recruitment and retention are vital to ensuring a workforce capable of delivering needed health care services, retention is ultimately the best recruitment strategy. Health care organizations—service and education—must develop workplaces that reward and challenge nurses, workplaces that support nurses in their goal of directing and delivering quality patient care. When employers build that type of workplace culture, nurses will remain and others will come.

Nurse retention improves the quality of health care. Numerous studies conducted in magnet hospitals demonstrate positive correlations between attraction and retention of professional nurses and quality patient care (McClure & Hinshaw, 2002). Studies also find that higher nurse-to-patient ratios improve morbidity and mortality rates and that too few nurses may increase health care costs (Aiken & Sloane, 1997; Aiken, Clarke, Sloane, Sochalski, & Silber, 2002).

Retaining nurses makes good business sense. Replacement costs for staff nurses are estimated at $50,000 each (Cohen & Sherrod, 2003), and considering additional expertise such as a critical care experience, costs may run $64,000 or more (Health Care Advisory Board, 2000a). Low turnover provides significant workforce development savings that can be redirected to improving patient care or the workplace environment.

In nursing education programs, faculty shortages are limiting program enrollments (American Association of Colleges of Nursing, 2004b). A study released by the Southern Regional Education Board (2002) documented a serious nursing faculty shortage in 16 states and reported a need for strategies to recruit and retain nursing faculty.

Creating a workplace environment that fosters retention requires serious thought and planning. Rome wasn't created in a day, and neither are productive retention programs. Development of a system for measuring retention is a must. Tracking unit and organizational vacancy rates, turnover rates, average tenure of employed nurses, average tenure of nurses who resign, and other measures can provide important information about your progress. Age analysis of nurses on various departments can assist agencies in proactively planning to refill vacancies caused by retirements. Establish accountability for retention processes through a retention/recruitment committee, nurse executive, nurse manager, or at the individual employee level.

Retention programs need to consider a number of factors that influence a nurse's decision to remain in or leave an organization, such as intense workload, lack of scheduling flexibility, low compensation, lack of continuing education, and little or no opportunity for career growth (American Organization of Nurse Executives, 2000; Health Care Advisory Board, 2000b; Mercer, 1999). Systematic feedback through nurse satisfaction surveys, exit interviews, and individual manager-nurse coaching interviews can provide additional issues for workplace improvement.

WORKFORCE RETENTION

While employers must retain enough nurses to deliver health care services, communities have an expressed interest in ensuring that there are enough direct care nurses, nurse managers, and nurse educators to provide for the evolving health needs of their citizens. Improving workplace cultures and environments can definitely influence choices of nurses to leave or remain in the nursing profession.

Communities must pay close attention to numbers of nurses considering leaving the profession. Already, studies are reporting that nurses demonstrate greater job dissatisfaction and emotional exhaustion when they are given responsibility for more patients than they can safely care for (Aiken, Sloane, Sochalski, & Silber, 2002). One study reports that as many as 30% of hospital nurses under the age of 30 plan to leave their current job (Aiken et al., 2001). Another reports that as many as 20% plan to remove themselves from direct-patient care responsibilities within the next five years (Peter D. Hart Research Associates, 2001). Research is needed to determine what is driving these nurses away. We'll need to look at creative strategies to retain nurses in the nursing profession.

WORKPLACE RECRUITMENT

Along with creating a positive, attractive work environment, employers must strengthen their employee pipeline with creative recruitment strategies. Recruit proactively. Position your facility as the "employer of choice" in your region. Deliver excellent health care and educational services, and get involved in your community.

You'll want to use traditional recruitment methods such as advertising in local newspapers, magazines, networks, etc. Internet advertising is cost effective, and more and more nurses are looking for jobs using electronic media. Maximize advertising reach and penetration. In other words, don't invest your entire recruitment budget on one advertisement you think nurses might see. Instead, invest in a number of advertisements and different locations or media that you know many nurses frequent.

Equip your nurses to serve as organizational ambassadors. Provide courses on public speaking and seek opportunities for them to teach health promotion and prevention courses to community groups or serve as resources or speakers on local radio or TV talk shows. Develop relationships with local radio, TV, and newspaper health care reporters and offer assistance and expertise.

Health care employers and schools of nursing should work together to establish relationships between students and potential employer. Employers might participate in open houses and career fairs. Schedule school visits and provide pizza for student-sponsored events throughout the year. Advertise in school-related publications or a student association magazine or newsletter. Host a senior reception a few months prior to graduation, or sponsor the pinning ceremony. Staff nurses might provide guest lectures or share their expertise as a professional mentor. Some hospitals are funding faculty positions, or even sharing their staff as faculty with local schools of nursing. Internship and externship programs have also been a successful strategy for developing relationships with nursing students.

Health care employers and schools of nursing should be partnering to address the rising demand for nurses. Nurse educational programs are the primary renewable resource for nurses in the community, and health care employers are where the jobs are located. Staff nurses should work closely with faculty to provide stellar clinical experiences. Scholarship programs should transition smoothly from the workplace setting to educational programs. To address rising nurse demand, both must plan creatively to develop and offer evening and weekend, on-site, online, and/or accelerated program options.

WORKFORCE RECRUITMENT

Even if all nurses choose to remain in nursing, we can expect a mass exodus within the next 10 years as baby-boomer nurses begin to retire. The average age of registered nurses is mid-40s and among faculty, mid-50s. As large numbers of nurses retire, demand for health care services is expected to dramatically increase as the boomer generation reaches their 60s, 70s, and 80s the golden age of health care service consumption.

Traditionally, people choose nursing because they want to "help people" or "make a difference in people's lives." For many years, if you were a woman and planned to attend college, the socially acceptable role was that of teacher or nurse. It is not surprising that U.S. registered nurses are 94.6% female and 86.6% white (USDHHS, BHPr Division of Nursing, 2002). Health care delivery organizations and schools of nursing must partner to provide a positive and inclusive image of nursing careers. We must develop creative recruitment strategies that focus on men, people of color, and other diverse student populations.

Some communities are already joining the effort. The community of Winston-Salem, North Carolina has established a healthcare roundtable to look at health care workforce solutions. The chamber of commerce heads the group, and partners include schools of nursing, hospitals, long-term care facilities, home health agencies, the area health education center, and representatives from local school systems. Four local hospitals are working together to provide a strategic regional marketing campaign to attract middle and high school youth to health care careers. Long-term recruitment strategies will need to target youth, displaced workers, individuals dissatisfied with their current career, and even older and retiring workers.

Employers and schools of nursing need to work closely with groups already positioned to increase health career awareness among individuals and groups. You may want to host a program that provides required educational credits for career counselors and career-explorer teachers in middle and high schools to inform them of the excitement, the decision-making power, the challenges, and the rewards of a nursing or health care career. Serve as an advisor for local health occupations education and assist in setting up observational experiences. Volunteer your organization to host students in job-shadowing experiences. Assist a local high school to develop a health sciences academy, which can provide additional resources to assist youth to jump-start a health care career. Establish a youth volunteer program or summer camp to expose youth to health care careers.

Recruitment and retention strategies are vital components of nurse workforce development. Due to increasing nurse demand in a complex and ever-changing health care arena, we must intensify efforts to develop innovative models for attracting and retaining nurses. And even when organizations have all positions filled, recruitment and retention processes will need to be systematically and continuously implemented. Consider the following examples related to workforce development.

EXEMPLAR #1—RECRUITMENT AND RETENTION INITIATIVES AT THE NORTH CAROLINA CENTER FOR NURSING (NCCN)

There are two distinct recruitment and retention activities carried out in the nursing community. Efforts to fill existing positions and keep current staff in individual health care agencies represent one type of recruitment and retention activity. The other is the replenishing of the nursing workforce and keeping nurses in the profession once they enter. The latter aspects of recruitment and retention are the focus of nursing workforce centers.

"Nursing: The Power to Make a Difference" Recruitment Campaign

Hemsley-Brown and Foskett (1999) identified that young people made career choices based on personal interest, enjoyment, and a desire to help people. In addition, they found that as early as sixth grade, young people would eliminate potential professions they did not view as positive even when they did not know in which career direction they would head. These decisions were often based on inaccurate perceptions formed from limited understanding of the lowest levels of a profession's activity. In other words these young people made decisions about a nursing career based on their perceptions of the work of nursing assistants. Those who chose nursing generally had personal contact with a nurse. The North Carolina Center for Nursing (NCCN) replicated this English study in urban and rural areas in North Carolina and found similar results across the state. Staiger, Auerbach, and Buerhaus (2000) reported that between 1973 and 2000, 40% fewer college freshmen indicate nursing as their top career choice as new opportunities opened to women in careers that were previously male dominated. Bednash (2000) reported that for five years in a row, nursing education programs across the United States experienced declining enrollments. Application of the nursing supply model by NCCN (Schmid & Lacey, 2000) predicted a coming nursing shortage in North Carolina. It was obvious that interest in nursing would have to be rekindled in those groups who in the past chose nursing as a primary career and that those groups who have been underrepresented in the nursing workforce needed to be introduced to nursing as a potential career choice.

Increasing the number of students choosing nursing and increasing the diversity of the nursing workforce required new thinking in the area of workforce recruitment. Nursing as a career needed to be made attractive again to students who in the past chose nursing, but it also needed to be inviting to the other groups of students who never considered nursing. Much has been written about the small size of the potential worker pool available from the generation known as Gen X. The low birthrate for Gen X has resulted in few new workers and heavy competition for each worker by all professions. Most members of this generation have made their initial career choice and entered the workforce. Some may choose nursing later as a second career, but they are not likely to be a significant source to replenish or grow the nursing workforce.

Generational researchers Zemke, Raines, and Filipczak (2000) reported on changes expected in the "Nexter" generation, those born after 1984. This generation will have a population close in numbers to the boomer generation. The defining characteristics of the nexter generation include civic-mindedness, optimism, confidence, technology driven, independence in work but team oriented, diverse, self-assured, seeking leadership opportunities, family oriented, and a desire to enjoy work. This generation really wants to "make a difference." If ever a generation could find fulfillment in a nursing career, this generation is it. They just need accurate and positive information on which to base their perceptions about nursing. Persistent stereotypes needed to be broken for males and underrepresented minority groups to increase interest and consideration of nursing as a career option.

These data were used to guide the development of NCCN's award-winning youth campaign, "Nursing: The Power to Make a Difference." This campaign was designed to provide nexters a positive and accurate look at nursing and to show the diversity of the work and workforce before young students are socialized to choose other careers. The campaign, developed in association with the Benard Hodes Group, is multifaceted and includes a dedicated Web page, high-powered video, a high-gloss brochure, age-appropriate posters, colorful pencils, ambassador cards, a dedicated group of nurse speakers, and a panel of "Power Nurses." For elementary age students, the campaign has coloring sheets and stickers about nursing.

A video, *Be the Difference,* is the anchor of the campaign targeted toward middle and high school students. The video explores nursing careers through the eyes of a young African-American female. Her decision to examine nursing is initiated by her observations of the level of job satisfaction she sees in her aunt, a home health nurse. Taking her aunt's advice, she volunteers at a local hospital. Through her volunteer work she is introduced to the varied roles of nurses both in and out of the hospital. The video runs 12 minutes and includes interviews with representatives of the nursing community at large and showcases ethnic, gender, and cultural groups that make up the nursing workforce. The challenge and difficulty of the journey to become a nurse is presented and several nurses discuss the positive aspects of nurse education. The campaign is centered around elements of nursing that would be attractive to the nexter generation. The general categories include the variety of work and workplace, powerful impact on lives, job security, flexibility, and job satisfaction in nursing. The video ends with the young student talking about how nursing matches her desire for a career that makes a difference in people's lives and work that is exciting. She refers anyone who wants to "make a difference" to the NCCN Website for additional information.

The video and other campaign materials were distributed to every public school, school nurse, and public library in North Carolina and were made available to other states for purchase. NCCN also provides copies of the video to nurses speaking to middle and high school groups. It is a powerful way to begin a discussion on nursing in a school or public setting.

Numerous campaign resources for speakers are available for download from the NCCN Web-site, including fact sheets about nursing and a PowerPoint presentation. Other campaign materials were designed to complement the video and get the message in students' hands. The brochure is dominated by eye-catching pictures of various nurses in different settings that depict the general categories used in the video. The brochures are given as handouts in each middle and high school presentation and at local career fairs. Bright purple pencils labeled with the NCCN Web-site URL are given to every age group. Stickers with logos are given to young children along with coloring sheets about nursing. Four age-appropriate posters were developed and sent to guidance counselors, career exploration teachers, and school nurses to mount on their walls. These posters are occasionally given out to students as prizes during drawings at large career-day events.

Ambassador cards were designed for nurses who volunteer as speakers. The size of a normal business card, these cards carry the campaign logos, colors, and photos. In addition there are talking points printed on the back of the card to remind the speaker about how to present nursing to young people. "Power nurses" write their nursing stories and describe their current work. Nurses provide an e-mail address, providing students with access to a nurse who can answer pertinent questions.

Other workforce recruitment programs developed by the NCCN include the Nurse Exploration Patch Program and the Health Care Careers book covers. Further information about the "Nursing: The Power to Make a Difference" campaign can be found on the student pages of the NCCN Web-site (http://www.nurseNC.org) or by contacting the North Carolina Center for Nursing.

North Carolina Institute for Nursing Excellence

Retention of the nursing workforce is another major program area for the nursing workforce centers. Most hiring agencies have some plan or program intended to retain their current nursing workforce. Like recruitment, the retention activities of nursing workforce centers focus on keeping nurses active in the nursing workforce. Traditionally, for many nurses the only advancement or reward for excellence was to assume a position removed from direct patient care activities.

The Institute for Nursing Excellence (INE) is a one-week professional development program designed to reward and revitalize outstanding direct care registered nurses. Excellent nurses, selected through a competitive process, attend a retreat (at the coast or in the mountains of North Carolina) for a week of professional and personal development. Employers must agree to grant administrative leave for selected nurses to attend the INE, but there are no registration costs for participants because the institute is funded by state dollars and private contributions.

Initially established as a biennial program, the INE was conducted in odd-numbered years for the past 10 years. Beginning in 2004, the program became an annual event. The stated purposes for the INE are to reward outstanding nurses, encourage excellent nurses to remain in the profession, develop leadership capacity in nurses of excellence, and enhance nurses' ability to be role models and attract others into nursing. The criteria for selection include full-time work status in North Carolina, a minimum of three years of experience as a registered nurse, and at least 50% of work time providing direct nursing care.

Institute applications are accepted for six months before the INE. Individual nurses, nurse supervisors, or clients can make nominations. Each nominee must submit a portfolio that includes statements from peers, supervisors, and clients that testify to the excellent status of the nominee. Hiring agencies are required to attest to the fact that at least 50% of the nominee's work time is in direct patient care. Each portfolio is blind reviewed by three members of the INE selection committee, which is made up of nursing leaders from across the state, including previous INE participants, staff nurses, nursing educators, nurse executives, and advanced practice nurses. The combined scores for each nominee are presented to the entire committee and the committee makes the final selections in a half-day meeting held at the center for nursing. Once INE nurses are selected, NCCN promotes their recognition through letters, press releases, and direct contact with the nurses' employing agencies.

The INE participants arrive at the retreat center for a continental breakfast and introductions on Monday morning and remain through lunch on Friday. Each day has three educational sessions and three to five hours of reflection time. Programs address critical nursing and leadership issues pertinent to the direct care registered nurse. Topics include cultural diversity, nursing involvement in public policy, using media, writing for publication, managing change, learning styles, workplace empowerment, sustaining a passion for nursing, North Carolina nursing history, team-building, networking, and understanding personality profiles using Myers-Briggs type indicators. State and national speakers are contracted as presenters. In addition to the serious aspects of personal and professional development, the week incorporates fun. In fact, speakers are evaluated on the elements of fun included in their presentations.

The INE classes are not passive. Presenters engage the nurses in serious dialogue while they draw pictures, play with soap bubbles, build towers, and write their own stories or songs to increase the personal learning. The INE participants are also required to get to know each other. By the second night, every member of the group is expected to be able to introduce any other member at the drop of a hat.

At the end of the week, nursing leaders from across the state join the INE participants for a recognition ceremony in which each participant receives an INE lapel pin and a certificate of completion. The nursing leaders offer words of praise, encouragement, and gratitude to the INE nurses. These presentations are followed by a gala luncheon to end the week. The NC center for nursing sends a press release with a photo to the newspapers of the participant's choice and also includes all INE alumni in a nursing excellence directory that is distributed to North Carolina schools, media outlets, and legislators.

Over 300 exemplary direct care nurses have been recognized through the INE program. These nurses differentiate themselves as clinical experts and identify themselves as a fraternity of sorts. They share a common history with every other INE graduate, regardless of their INE class, and view each other as peers and an extended professional network. The INE graduates are honored each year with a reception during the North Carolina center for nursing's annual advisory council meeting. After 15 successful years, the INE is going through evaluation and revision. The recruitment and retention pages of the NCCN Web-site (http://www.nurseNC.org) will have additional information about the revisions as they occur as well as coverage and photographs of the most recent INE week.

EXEMPLAR #2—A CASE FOR COLLABORATION RELATED TO DEVELOPMENT OF THE NURSING WORKFORCE IN INDIANA

Nursing 2000 is an innovative model of collaboration between nursing service and nursing education serving a 10-county area in central Indiana. Founded 14 years ago, the organization exists for the promotion and support of registered nursing careers at all levels of development to positively impact future health care resources. Organizational outcomes are the result of individuals and groups working together to advance nursing.

Leadership for the organization is a concerted effort. An 8-member executive board of nurse executive and dean/director representatives provides direction and vision. A 30-member advisory board with representatives from health care facilities, schools of nursing, and professional nursing associations develops and evaluates programs. Two hundred volunteers carry out the activities of Nursing 2000. The staff who support the volunteers include an executive director, a part-time program facilitator, an administrative assistant, and a part-time staff assistant. Indianapolis regional health care facilities and schools of nursing financially support Nursing 2000. Program development has been supplemented in part by grants.

Nursing 2000 represents one long-term solution to impact the development of a well-educated nursing workforce at the local level. Nursing 2000 goal setting has three essential assumptions that serve as the focus for collaboration: the development of the educational pipeline; nursing educational mobility to prepare nurses for roles in direct care, advanced practice, education, and research; and community relationship building to form working alliances. The assumptions are inherent in the goals of the organization (Table 8.1).

Development of the Pipeline

Nursing 2000 members addressed pipeline development as the initial focus of collaboration. Programs and activities were targeted at elementary, middle, and high school students, as well as adult

TABLE 8.1   Goals of Nursing 2000

* Impact the education of nurses through collaboration between nursing service and education.
* Present nursing as a rewarding and dynamic career in demand.
* Support nurses in educational mobility and clinical practice to advance nursing careers.
* Recruit a diverse student body reflective of the regional population.
* Attract students into nursing who have demonstrated the potential academic abilities that will lead to a successful career in nursing.
* Reflect a positive image of nursing to the public.

learner students such as individuals interested in a second college degree. Career materials to promote nursing as a dynamic and rewarding career were created for use in classroom presentations, career fairs, community seminars, and career counseling. An informational Web-site was created to access career materials and link visitors to career resources (Table 8.2).

Additional career tools were created to promote and educate the public about nursing careers. A seven-minute videotape, *Nursing Today and Beyond 2000,* presents the opportunities, academic preparation, and rewards in nursing. The videotape was distributed to community intermediate and secondary schools and public libraries in central Indiana. A poster, "Nursing is AMAZING: Challenge Yourself, Change Lives, Choose Nursing," was created to depict current practice roles. The poster was disseminated to school nurses throughout the state for display in their offices. A newsletter, *Future Focus in Nursing,* was published three times per year. Targeted to middle and high school counselors, the newsletter features nursing specialties, nursing profiles, the demand for nursing, and Nursing 2000 programs.

The flagship of the Nursing 2000 model quickly became the shadow program, A Day in the Life of a Nurse. The structured program, targeted to high school students, facilitated RN role modeling, academic counseling, counselor rapport, parental contact, and school of nursing contacts, and also enhanced linkages between the health care community and high schools. Based on evaluative surveys conducted by Nursing 2000 leadership and Indiana University School of Nursing, the program was beneficial to students as a career exploration experience. A 22-item, multiple-choice survey, Choosing a Career in Nursing, was mailed (in two consecutive

TABLE 8.2   Career Materials Accessible on Nursing 2000 Web-Site

- A Career in Registered Nursing
- Schools of Nursing in Indiana
- Specialties in the Career of Registered Nursing
- Nursing Organization Resource List
- Volunteer Opportunities in Affiliated Hospitals
- Financial Aid Resource
- RN Educational Mobility Guide
- LPN to RN Mobility Guide
- Guide to Specialty Certification in the Career of Registered Nursing

years) to 625 graduating high school seniors who had participated in the shadow program as sophomores, juniors, or seniors. The purpose of the survey was to examine factors that affected participants' decision to pursue nursing as a career. The combined response rate was 27%. The respondents represented 36 different Indiana high schools spread across an eight-county Nursing 2000 service area. Findings, depicted in Figure 8.1, revealed participants made the decision to pursue nursing sometime between the 10th and 12th grades (Briggs, Merk, & Mitchell, 2003). Participants were influenced most often by friends and family members in the nursing profession. High school teachers and a personal experience with a nurse also had influence over the participants' decision to pursue nursing (see Table 8.3).

Other factors also impacted respondents' decision to pursue nursing. Seventy-five percent found the shadow program as moderately to highly influential in their decision to choose nursing (Briggs, Merk, & Mitchell, 2003). "Fifty-three percent of the respondents indicated observing a nurse at work influenced their actual decision to pursue nursing. This was followed by observing a sick family member or friend (32%); working or volunteering in a healthcare setting (28%); watching TV or movies that featured nurses (26%); personal experiences as a patient (22%); reading books or stories about nurses or nursing (10%); and being a member in a career club that stressed science, math, or health (8%)" (Briggs, Merk, & Mitchell, 2003, p. 116).

In annual surveys sent to graduating high school seniors, respondents report an increasing enrollment in nursing school from 57% in 1999 to 70% in 2002 (Nursing 2000, 2002). In a survey sent to 1,598 nursing students enrolled in affiliated nursing schools, A

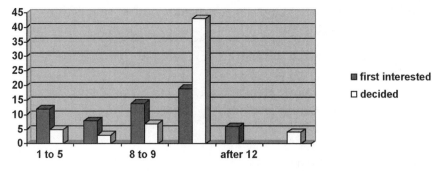

FIGURE 8.1   Timing of career decisions (N = 165).
Note: Collaboration for the Promotion of Nursing (p. 114), by L. Briggs, S. E. Merck, and B. Mitchell, 2003, Indianapolis, IN: Sigma Theta Tau International. Copyright 2003 by Sigma Theta Tau International. Reprinted with permission.

Day in the Life of a Nurse shadow program was found to be statistically significant at the p value of .0001 as influential in choice of careers (Wilson & Mitchell, 1999, pp. 59–60). Thus, evaluative surveys reflect that the program is an effective career exploration program based on nursing students' feedback prior to enrollment and postenrollment in the nursing major.

Collaboration between nursing service and education was enhanced as age-based programs were developed and evaluated. Recruitment initiatives and the creation of opportunities for career decision making became the foundation for collaboration.

Supporting Educational Mobility

Collaboration is essential to support educational mobility. Three career mobility seminars were planned to reach out to the community. The first seminar, Nursing Now—A First Look at Nursing as a Career, is structured for both the traditional student and the adult learner. The seminar presents the demand for nursing at all levels of preparation, and an interactive RN panel presents nursing role diversity. Representatives and opportunities from schools of nursing are available as resources pre- and postseminar. Previous participants in the shadow program who are currently junior or senior high school students are invited, as are their parents. A second seminar, Spotlight on Reentry, reaches out to the inactive registered nurse. The program presents the role of the RN in the current health care environment, refresher course opportunities, and accessing reentry into the job market. Registered nurses discuss their experiences as

TABLE 8.3   People of Influence

(N = 165)

Categories	Percentage of respondents
Friend/neighbor pursing nursing as a career	24%
Family member a nurse	22%
High school teacher	15%
Nurse who cared for me	15%
Other: Non-nurse family members	11%
High school counselor	10%
Recruiter/counselor from a nursing program	5%
Other: experience observing nursing care	3%
College/university recruiter	2%

Note: From *Collaboration for the Promotion of Nursing* (p. 114), by L. Briggs, S. E. Merck, and B. Mitchell, 2003, Indianapolis, IN: Sigma Theta Tau International. Copyright 2003 by Sigma Theta Tau International. Reprinted with permission.

they have successfully reentered the workplace. A third seminar, Advanced Roles in Nursing—Opportunities and Challenges, provides a collegial exchange regarding advanced practice. A panel of experts discusses the expectations and responsibilities of various advanced nursing practice roles. Graduate nursing program representatives are present as resources.

Career materials were created to support nurses as they explored options to advance their educational preparation. An educational mobility guide provides a resource for the registered nurse exploring RN-BSN, RN-MSN, MSN, and PhD nursing educational programs in Indiana. A second guide serves as a resource for nursing certification and a third was created for the licensed practical nurse pursuing a career as a registered nurse (Briggs, Merk, & Mitchell, 2003).

An annual scholarship benefit was established to assist undergraduate and graduate students enrolled in a nursing major with their financial commitments. The benefit receives support from health care facilities, corporations, nursing organizations, friends, and colleagues. The volunteer effort has resulted in $328,000 cumulative proceeds benefiting 397 students in the form of nursing scholarships (Nursing 2000, 2003). The benefit supports nursing students at all levels of development and degrees and fosters educational access from entry level to advanced degrees.

As the interdependency among the programs increased, the viability and value of the programs increased. Collaboration was broadened across the community.

Community Building

Community building is essential to provide responsive programs and working alliances. At a time of increased expectations for patient care delivery when the supply and educational mix of nursing resources are underrepresented, concerted solutions are needed in the broader community (U.S. Government Accounting Office, 2001). In 2001, two initiatives were concurrently launched: replicating the Nursing 2000 model, adapted to unique differences, in another region of the state, and facilitating a statewide nursing workforce summit.

A Helene Fuld Trust Grant was received to replicate the Nursing 2000 model in another region of the state based on regional uniqueness. A written guide was developed of the Nursing 2000 model including primary programs and activities of the organization that evolved into a book, *Collaboration for the Promotion of Nursing,* published by Sigma Theta Tau International (Briggs, Merk, & Mitchell, 2003). Due to the exemplary leadership of nursing service and nursing education leaders in north central Indiana, the Nursing 2000 model was adapted to a four-county region. The organization became Nursing 2000 North Central, Inc.

The impact of regional programs becomes greater when in synchrony with concerted, statewide efforts. Regional programs are essential for workforce development because they extend into the local community and serve as integral components of statewide workforce development. Nursing 2000 and Nursing 2000 North Central are part of the Indiana Nursing Workforce Development Coalition (INWDC), which includes Indiana health care providers, nursing organizations, nurse educators, nurse leaders, and stakeholders working to systematically address the nursing supply needs in the state.

The Indiana Nursing Workforce Development Coalition evolved from a 2001 nursing shortage summit meeting. The statewide planning committee included representatives from the Indiana Association of Homes and Services for the Aging, Indiana Organization of Nurse Executives, Indiana Health Care Association, Indiana Hospital and Health Association, Indiana Schools of Nursing, Indiana State Nurses Association, VHA Central, and Nursing 2000 Vice Presidents and Deans Forum. The summit had 150 attendees, representing health care, education, nursing organizations, and policy makers attended (Briggs, Merk, & Mitchell, 2003, pp. 132–133). An action plan, steering committee, and workgroups evolved from the summit. The workgroups addressed five areas: (1) nursing as an economic issue for the state; (2) a consistent message for nursing in Indiana; (3) nursing service and education partnerships; (4) data, information, and communication; and (5) infrastructure to support and sustain the work. The outcomes included a white paper, *The Nursing Workforce Shortage in Indiana-Current Status and Future Trends;* a Web-site, (http://www.indiananursingworkforce.org); regional summits in the northwest and southwest part of the state; a statewide survey on nursing student enrollments/graduations and faculty vacancies/projected needs; a faculty pool project pilot to maximize faculty resources; distribution of Indiana data from benchmarking surveys on registered nurse vacancies and health care workforce projections from gap analysis data; testimony to policy makers on nursing workforce needs; and procurement of minimal financial support to maintain the work until sustaining funding sources could be obtained.

Nursing and health care leaders have remained committed to nursing workforce development. The work requires dedicated resources to coordinate the steering committee and workgroup chairpersons, which has, to date, been performed as a volunteer and in-kind effort. Great strides have been made in sharing and networking across the state. The movement in the state has concurrently embraced regional uniqueness and the collective impact of the Indiana Nursing Workforce Development Coalition. Collaboration leads to community relationship building. It is a magnetizing process from which working alliances emerge.

As a result of Nursing 2000's involvement in the Indiana Nursing Workforce Development Coalition and Nursing 2000 North Central, the impact of promoting the development of future nursing careers is greater. Its members strive to be responsive to the local, regional, and statewide community.

9

Sustainable Infrastructures: The Growth and Funding of State-Level Nursing Workforce Centers

Mary Lou Brunell, Rebecca Rice, Brenda Cleary, Ann Duncan, and Fran Roberts

As described in the first chapter, state nursing workforce entities have come into their own within the past few years. Fueled partly by the nursing shortage and through the coordinated efforts of the states and regions (funded and nonfunded by the Robert Wood Johnson Foundation) involved in Colleagues in Caring, these entities now number close to 40, if one counts all the states that have brought together coalitions around nursing workforce issues. This chapter describes the results of a survey conducted in spring 2003 to describe the current state of funded statewide nursing workforce centers. Following this discussion, four centers' structure, funding, and work are described.

A SURVEY OF THE CENTERS IN 2003

In spring 2003, as a result of a charge to the Florida Center for Nursing, we surveyed each of the 13 established statewide nursing workforce centers. The purpose of the survey was to describe the structure, funding, and activities of the centers in order to inform the Florida nursing center stakeholders. In addition, we thought that having this information would be useful for other states as they set out to create their own nursing workforce entities.

Using a self-developed survey tool, we interviewed by telephone each of the 13 center directors in February and March 2003. Survey participants included center directors from Alaska, Colorado, Connecticut, Florida, Iowa, Michigan, Mississippi, Nebraska, Oregon, North Carolina, South Dakota, Tennessee, and Vermont. The data were then analyzed using descriptive statistics.

Of the 13 centers surveyed, all but one were established in 2000 and 2001. The North Carolina Center was established in 1991. Boards of directors govern seven of the centers, and the others possess some sort of external group that advised the centers. The participating stakeholder groups and/or the legislature or governor appoint the board members.

All the centers operate with small staffs and on small budgets. In fact, nine do not employ specifically defined staff (the work was subsumed within the agency in which the centers are housed). Of those centers with defined staff, most staff are designated as part-time employees. Seven centers employ two to three full-time-equivalent staff. Centers operate on funds from a variety of sources, including the state, foundations, donations, license renewal fees, revenue-generating projects, and others. The total annual budgets for the centers range from less than $50,000 to over $500,000, with a bimodal distribution of three centers operating on $50,000–$100,000 and three at over $500,000.

The work of the centers focuses on meeting their charges as defined in their mission statements. Strategic planning for nursing workforce issues is central to the work of the centers. In addition, the majority of the state nursing workforce centers (10 of 13) focus their work on the evidence base for addressing workforce issues, dissemination of nursing workforce data to interested constituencies, the development and assessment of a nursing workforce to meet the health care needs of the citizens, and the development of incentive and recognition programs for nurses.

Working with nursing workforce data is pivotal to creating and maintaining the evidence base for nursing workforce issues. Nine centers describe their role with data as including serving as a clearinghouse, being identified as a source of data, and assisting with modification of data collection. The data task force of the Colleagues in Caring program had identified a minimum supply data set to which the CIC sites ascribed. This data set was widely disseminated to all the states requesting it. Of the 13 centers surveyed, at least 10 use the minimum supply data elements.

Finally, we asked the survey participants about the role that the centers play in communication of nursing workforce issues. The centers both convene meetings and serve as a conduit of information. Most frequently, the centers indicated they participate in meetings of stakeholder groups, advisory committees, task forces, regional and state forums, meetings with students and guidance counselors, and focus groups. In addition, the centers disseminate information about nursing workforce issues through their Web-sites, newsletters, and presentations.

Included in this chapter are examples from four centers. They are all different. For example, Arizona's Healthcare Institute includes nursing and allied health professions and is funded and housed at the Arizona Hospital and Healthcare Association. North Carolina, Florida, and Tennessee all have been formed by state legislative action and receive funding not only from the state but also from grants and other donations. Most have similar missions. Below, the four centers describe their structure and funding, their successes to date, and their lessons learned.

THE NORTH CAROLINA CENTER FOR NURSING (NCCN)

Creation and Funding of the NCCN

The creation of the NCCN was a visionary response to the nursing shortage of the late 1980s and a significant departure from the "quick fix" mentality that had typically shaped nurse workforce policy. North Carolina became the first state to fund an agency dedicated to ensuring adequate nursing resources to meet the health care needs of its citizens. The inception of the center for nursing was the culmination of three years of work by the North Carolina General Assembly and the Legislative Study Commission on Nursing. The Nursing Shortage Act of 1991 in GS (General Statute) 90-171.70 in Article 9F, Chapter 550 of the 1991 North Carolina General Assembly Session Laws, included the center's enabling legislation and can be found in Table 9.1.

The NCCN's state-appropriated funding has remained relatively consistent at $500,000 per annum. The center seeks to increase the total resource available each year by approximately 25% through external funds (grants and private contributions), bringing the annual budget to just over $600,000.

The board of directors provides broad oversight of the work of the North Carolina Center for Nursing, and the University of North Carolina Office of the President provides administrative support.

TABLE 9.1   Enabling Legislation Establishing the North Carolina Center for Nursing

There is established the North Carolina center for nursing to address issues of supply and demand for nursing, including issues of recruitment, retention, and utilization of nurse manpower resources. The General Assembly finds that the Center will repay the State's investment by providing an ongoing strategy for the allocation of the State's resources directed towards nursing. The primary goals for the Center shall be:

1. To develop a strategic statewide plan for nursing manpower in North Carolina by:
   a. Establishing and maintaining a database on nursing supply and demand in North Carolina, to include current supply and demand, and future projections; and
   b. Selecting priorities from the plan to be addressed.
2. To convene various groups representative of nurses, other health care providers, business and industry, consumers, legislators, and educators to:
   a. Review and comment on data analysis prepared for the Center;
   b. Recommend systemic changes, including strategies for implementation of recommended changes; and
   c. To evaluate and report the results of these efforts to the General Assembly and others.
3. To enhance and promote recognition, reward, and renewal activities for nurses in North Carolina by:
   a. Promoting continuation of Institutes for Nursing Excellence programs as piloted by the Area Health Education Centers in 1989–90 or similar options;
   b. Proposing and creating additional reward, recognition and renewal activities for nurses; and
   c. Promoting media and positive image-building efforts for nursing.

The North Carolina center for nursing shall be governed by a policy-setting board of directors. The Board shall consist of 16 members, with a simple majority of the Board being nurses representative of various practice areas. Other members shall include representatives of other health care professions, business and industry, health care providers, and consumers. The Board shall be appointed as follows:

1. Four members appointed by the General Assembly upon recommendation of the President Pro Tempore of the Senate, at least one of whom shall be a registered nurse and at least one other a representative of the hospital industry;
2. Four members appointed by the General Assembly upon the recommendation of the Speaker of the House of Representatives, at least one of whom shall be a registered nurse and at least one other a representative of the long-term care industry;

(continued)

TABLE 9.1   Enabling Legislation Establishing the North Carolina Center for Nursing *(Continued)*

3. Four members appointed by the Governor, two of whom shall be registered nurses; and
4. Four nurse educators, one of whom shall be appointed by the Board of Governors of The University of North Carolina, one other by the State Board of Community Colleges, one other by the North Carolina Association of Independent Colleges and Universities, and one by the Area Health Education Centers Program.

After the initial appointments expire, the terms of all the members shall be three years, with no member serving more than two consecutive terms.

The Board of Directors shall have the following powers and duties:

1. To employ the Executive Director;
2. To determine operational policy;
3. To elect a chairperson and officers, to serve two-year terms. The chairperson and officers may not succeed themselves;
4. To establish committees of the Board as needed;
5. To appoint a multidisciplinary advisory council for Input and advice on policy matters;
6. To implement the major functions of the center for nursing as established in the goals set out in this section; and
7. To seek and accept non-state funds for carrying out Center policy.

The General Assembly further finds that it is imperative that the State protect its investment and progress made in nursing efforts to date. The General Assembly finds that the North Carolina center for nursing is the appropriate means to do so. The Center shall have State budget support for its operations so that it may have adequate resources for the tasks the General Assembly has set out in this Article.

The six staff members of the center, currently consisting of the executive director; associate director for research, associate director for recruitment and retention, research associate, information and communications specialist, and administrative secretary, manage the day-to-day operations.

Meeting the Legislative Mandates

Goal 1—Strategic Statewide Plan

To meet the goal of developing a strategic statewide plan for nursing in North Carolina, the center for nursing:

- established and maintains a comprehensive database describing the existing supply of nurses
- assesses the demand for nurses throughout the state through surveys of nurse employers
- created the North Carolina Nurse Workforce Planning Model for bringing together nursing leaders from education and practice as well as professional organizations/agencies in North Carolina to shape nursing's preferred future, with funding from state hospitals, the Duke Endowment, and the Robert Wood Johnson Foundation
- sponsored a number of other workforce planning initiatives, including a future think tank, a statewide steering committee for articulation in nursing education (funded by the Helene Fuld Trust), and a task force on the nursing workforce, in conjunction with the North Carolina Institute of Medicine, the North Carolina Area Health Education Centers, the NC Nurses Association, and the NC Hospital Association and funded by the Duke Endowment.

Goal 2—Interdisciplinary Collaboration

The 16-member board of directors and the six center staff seek input from nurses, other health care providers, educators, representatives of business and industry, policy makers, and consumers to ensure strategic planning that meets the needs of all North Carolina citizens. The center convenes various groups to review findings and evaluate the policy implications. These groups include an advisory council and project advisory committees.

The center has a 50-member advisory council composed of leaders from across the state in nursing and health care, business and industry, education, the state general assembly, and consumer groups. The board of directors appoints the advisory council members. Working through the board of directors and advisory council, priorities are identified in a comprehensive report to the general assembly each biennium.

Project advisory committees provide guidance during project development and evaluation upon project completion. These committees are composed of a variety of stakeholders whose expertise lies in the projects' purposes.

Goal 3—Recognition, Reward, and Renewal

The NCCN has several statewide initiatives to promote nurse recruitment and retention, including the Institute for Nursing Excellence and a recruitment and retention grant program. Each is described below.

The Institute for Nursing Excellence (INE) is a statewide program that rewards outstanding direct care nurses, encourages them to remain in nursing, increases their leadership capabilities, and enhances their ability to be role models and attract others into the profession. A workshop and reunion for INE participants is provided annually to promote continued professional development. Glaxo Wellcome and the Gannett Foundation have been funding partners for the institute.

The center also publishes a directory of INE. The directory, updated annually, promotes recognition of nurses and their contributions to health care in North Carolina. The directory also provides education and health care systems, the media, and policy makers with information about the experience and expertise of institute participants.

The recruitment and retention grant program is funded by the state and offered biennially to support activities aimed at retention of expert nurses and nurse recruitment, particularly in specific specialties and for underrepresented minorities and geographic areas where the supply of nurses does not meet the demand. The grants provide agencies employing nurses with resources to develop and implement local programs for promoting and recognizing nursing excellence.

In 1999, the NCCN embarked on a recruitment campaign, Nursing: The Power to Make a Difference. In building this campaign, the center held focus groups to aid in the development of media and Internet applications depicting nursing as a viable and attractive career option. Once launched, the campaign aired televised and radio public service announcements statewide. Thousands of young people were asked to "consider nursing" by volunteers representing the center for nursing at the annual state fair. Talking points for how to interest kids in nursing were also widely distributed. Newspaper inserts profiling nursing roles are being distributed throughout the state. A nursing exploration patch program was developed for the Girl Scouts, Boy Scouts, and Career Explorer programs, in collaboration with the North Carolina Association of Nursing Students. The center is continually enhancing its Web-site (http://www.nurseNC.org) to serve as a clearinghouse for state nursing career information to be used by guidance counselors, teachers, students, and the public. Table 9.2 depicts the deliverables from the campaign.

TABLE 9.2   North Carolina Recruitment Campaign Deliverables

Nursing: The Power to Make A Difference

- TV and radio public service announcements
- "Newspapers in Education" program
- Award-winning nursing video available to all state schools
- "Nursing in North Carolina" Internet site
- "Nursing Exploration" patch program
- Elementary school poster
- Middle/high school posters
- Book cover project, promoting nursing and other health careers, underwritten by Eli Lilly
- "Talk with Kids about Nursing" ambassador cards
- Fact sheets (in English and Spanish) and information packets for school counselors and health occupations teachers

Lessons Learned

The center for nursing serves all stakeholders concerned with North Carolina's nursing workforce, and the ultimate stakeholders are the citizens of the state. We have in place a well-developed research agenda for monitoring nursing supply and demand in North Carolina. Based on secondary analysis of licensure data, we have studied trends in nurse supply data dating back to 1982, which we are now augmenting with sample surveys of North Carolina nurses. We measure demand by means of a statewide survey of nurse employers. We know that the growth of RN full-time equivalents has exceeded the growth of the population in general and that vacancy rates are lower than those of other states with comparative data. We have an active database of nearly 500 Institute for Nursing Excellence participants, all of whom have been retained in nursing and cite the institute as a major factor. The recruitment and retention grant program has attracted matching funds of $2.38 for every $1 of state funds invested for nurse recruitment and retention programs at the agency level. Staying viable means connecting with all the stakeholders in nursing care.

The creation of the NCCN was a pioneering effort of the general assembly back in 1991, requiring a long-range vision of nurse workforce planning as opposed to the quick fixes of the past. The NCCN is a visible commitment to the criticality of nursing resources and fulfills its mission by (1) providing objective information to health care providers, policy makers, and other stakeholders; (2) developing a strategic planning mechanism for nursing resources in North Carolina; and (3) promoting recruitment and retention by recognizing and rewarding excellence and ensuring recognition among nurse colleagues. The center is an exciting innovation, with resources allocated to developing long-term nursing workforce solutions. The NCCN constitutes an agency dedicated to providing leadership in pulling together various stakeholders in nurse work-force planning and policy. Actions taken by the center over the past 13 years have positioned North Carolina well in terms of addressing the evolving national and international nursing short-age. The fact that, based on the limited comparative data available, North Carolina is faring better than many states, has led to increas-ing interest in the center for nursing as a model for state nursing workforce initiatives.

TENNESSEE CENTER FOR NURSING (TCN)

Creation of the TCN

In fall 1995, Tennessee responded to a request for proposals issued by the Robert Wood Johnson Foundation for the Colleagues in Caring (CIC) program. The purpose of this program was to enhance regional and state collaboration and planning and to recommend actions to address issues and changes occurring in the United States in the nursing labor market. Drs. Patricia L. Smith and Nancy B. Moody submitted a proposal on behalf of East Tennessee State University and the Tennessee Department of Health (TDH). As part of the appli-cation process, collaborators pledged additional funds (in kind and cash) totaling $251,981. Tennessee was selected for funding and received an additional $199,891 from the Robert Wood Johnson Foundation. The grand total of funding from the Robert Wood Johnson Foundation and private contributors for the project over the three-year period June 1996 through December 1999 was $554,829.

The Tennessee initiative, dubbed the Tennessee Healthcare Consortium for Nursing (THCN), was led by the project codirectors and a staff composed of three directors of assessment and planning from the TDH (one from each of the three grand divisions of the state-east, middle, and west), three nursing education coordinators from the same grand divisions, and three ex-officio representatives from the TDH.

THCN membership included representatives from consumer and business organizations, the Tennessee General Assembly, state departments and regulatory boards, public and private nursing education programs, professional nursing organizations and foundations, related health care agencies and organizations, and members at large.

Robert Wood Johnson Foundation funding ended in December 1999. From January through July 2000, THCN was funded by donations from individuals and organizations throughout the state, and members expressed continuing commitment to sustain the consortium. THCN applied for and was awarded a grant from the BlueCross BlueShield Community Trust to employ a grant writer. Beginning in July 2000, the THCN entered into a one-year contract with BlueCross BlueShield of Tennessee (BCBST). This funding enabled THCN to employ an executive director and an administrative assistant on a half-time basis. Dr. Nancy B. Moody became the first executive director of the organization one month later, and the THCN office was relocated to the University of Tennessee at Knoxville. During the subsequent fiscal year, data were collected to meet the scope of services for the BCBST contract, and the organization reorganized as a 501{c}3 nonprofit charitable organization with the new name of Tennessee Center for Nursing (TCN), Inc. New bylaws were adopted, and THCN members became TCN board of directors. Semiannual meetings of the corporation were conducted, and several nursing research studies were produced.

In November 2000, the Tennessee Nurses Association unanimously supported a resolution that the Tennessee Board of Nursing enter into a contract with the TCN to establish a statewide center for nursing workforce planning and development. During the following session of the Tennessee General Assembly, legislation was enacted enabling the Tennessee Board of Nursing to enter into contracts with nonprofit statewide organizations for several reasons, including nursing workforce planning.

In spring 2001, the Tennessee Primary Care Association and TCN applied and were approved for a grant from the Health Resources Service Administration, Bureau of Health Professions that enabled TCN to establish a Web-site to make the TCN data and printed materials available in the public domain. In addition, the BSBST contract with TCN was extended from August 1, 2001, through July 31, 2002.

At the September 2001 Tennessee Board of Nursing meeting, the board voted to enter into a contract with the TCN, and a scope of services was developed that provided for TCN to serve as the research arm of the Tennessee Board of Nursing. The contract was executed to begin January 2002 and end 18 months later in June 2003. A search committee was established by the TCN board of directors to recruit and employ a full-time executive director. During the search for a full-time executive director, the TCN entered into a contract with Lincoln Memorial University for interim services of its president, Dr. Nancy B. Moody, and for 10% of the university's administrative staff time.

Center Infrastructure

A full-time executive director, Ann P. Duncan, was employed in June 2002, and the TCN office was relocated to Nashville, Tennessee. As a nonprofit corporation chartered for business in the state, the TCN was no longer a contractual entity under the aegis of a state university. Administrative procedures for employing staff had to be developed, and payroll, banking, and other business operations had to be established. Professional services for legal, certified public accounting, and information technology were obtained. Company membership in a group health plan was started and, subsequent to arranging for payroll services, a full-time administrative assistant was employed.

The Tennessee Board of Nursing renewed the contract with the TCN for a two-year period from July 1, 2003, to June 31, 2005. The TCN continues to seek additional funding from contributions and grants.

The mission of the TCN is as follows:

> To develop a sustainable process through community partner-ships to guide the ongoing development of a nursing workforce appropriately educated, geographically distributed, and with the capacity to adapt to change and meet the health care needs of Tennesseans.

To implement its mission, TCN activities are organized by five board committees: policy and public relations, recruitment and retention, research, statewide educational planning, and strategic planning.

Lessons Learned

The TCN journey has evolved, changing its name, structure, and financing since its initial inception in 1996. However, the commit-ment of the stakeholders has been steady and strong. Here is what we've learned.

Success of a nursing workforce center is directly proportional to the diversity of the governing body. The board of the Tennessee Center for Nursing is not exclusively nurses. Rather, it is composed of individuals representing a broad spectrum of associations, corporations, agencies, departments, universities, and the legislature. When a nursing workforce issue needs the support of these organizations, they have been "at the table." Having been involved in the process, they understand the issue and can assist in following through with the needed action within their organization.

There will never be enough money. Nursing workforce issues have to addressed using new approaches and strategies. There will never be enough money to solve the nursing shortage by doing "business as usual."

There are no quick fixes or "magic bullets" for solving nursing workforce issues. It is essential to have continuing commitment from the stakeholders to work toward future solutions. Being proactive by identifying current and emerging problems, prioritizing strategic action, and asking "how are we going to effect a positive change" rather than "why is it this way" are critical to the ongoing work.

Stay on message. Nursing workforce centers need to become the recognized, credible source for clear, concise, timely, and accurate information about nursing workforce issues to media, higher education, other professionals, and the nursing profession. The information and recommendations must be data driven, evidence based, and specific to the state. Although national and regional data are important, local data are what capture the attention and action of the center's constituency. Developing the key messages and repeatedly delivering them to targeted audiences is essential in building awareness and action.

FLORIDA CENTER FOR NURSING (FCN)

Creation of the FCN

As a result of collaboration and professional commitment from statewide nursing leaders, during its 2001 session the Florida Legislature passed statute 464.0195 establishing the FCN. The FCN was created primarily through the advocacy efforts of a coalition of nursing organizations, including the Florida Nurses Association (FNA), the Florida Organization of Nurse Executives (FONE), the Florida Deans and Directors (D&D), and the Florida Hospital

Association (FHA). In March 2001, FNA held a legislative summit bringing together leadership from the FONE, the D&D, and the FHA. At this event, the concept of the FCN was formalized. During the legislative session, FNA and FHA presented the concept to the state legislature. Incredibly, in one legislative session the language was drafted and the bill passed. The cohesive commitment among all these stakeholder organizations to address the nursing shortage in Florida clearly influenced the outcome. To propose, draft, and pass statutory language establishing a center during the same legislative session is truly uncommon and speaks to the strength of nursing when unified.

The statute establishing the FCN defines its purpose:

> To address issues of supply and demand for nursing, including issues of recruitment, retention, and utilization of nurse workforce resources. The Legislature finds that the Center will repay the state's investment by providing an ongoing strategy for the allocation of the state's resources directed towards nursing (Florida Center for Nursing, 2001).

By statute, the FCN goals address collecting and analyzing nursing workforce data, developing and disseminating a strategic plan for nursing, developing and implementing reward and recognition activities for nurses, promoting nursing excellence programs, image building, and recruiting into the profession. The FCN is further charged to convene various stakeholder groups to review and comment on nursing workforce data and to recommend systemic changes that will improve the recruitment and retention of nurses in Florida. The FCN reports on the results of its work to the state legislature and others as determined by the legislature.

A companion legislative statute (§ 464.0196, 2001) set the structure for the FCN. The FCN is governed by a policy-setting board of directors, whose membership is specified according to the statute. Board members must include representatives from the FNA, the FHA, the FONE, and associate and baccalaureate programs of nursing education. The governor appoints all members and receives recommendations from the state senate, house of representatives, and board of education.

The FCN board employs the executive director, determines operational policy, elects its chair and officers, and establishes committees. The board also appoints a multidisciplinary advisory council for input on policy matters. The board may solicit and accept nonstate funds to sustain the work of the center.

Funding

Delayed by circumstances resulting from the September 11th terrorist attack, the FCN held its inaugural meeting on March 1, 2002. At that time, the University of Central Florida College of Health and Public Affairs (COHPA) was designated to house the FCN. Annually the university enters into a state contract to serve as fiscal agent for the FCN. For the first two years, the Florida Agency for Healthcare Administration held the contract for the FCN. Currently, the Florida Department of Health is the contracting agency.

The FCN has been funded as a nonrecurring line item in Florida's budget for each of its three years in the amount of $250,000. Because it is a nonrecurring item, the funding must be sought annually during the legislative session. Funding must appear in and be retained by the senate, the house, and the governor's budgets.

The effort to fund the FCN from state funds has been successful for each fiscal year of the center's existence to date. In reality, this is minimal funding, inadequate to meet the statutory mandates given the FCN. The center's funding accommodates the following:

1.0 full-time equivalent (FTE) for an executive director
0.5 FTE for an assistant director (new position in year 3)
1.0 FTE for an executive secretary
Temporary help and consultation
Expenses (equipment, office supplies, telephones, travel, computer support, etc.)
University indirect charge at 5%

Approximately 80% of the total budget is allocated to salaries and benefits. The university's charge for FCN use of human resources, office space, and other support is considerably less than charged for most contracts and grants.

During the 2002 Florida legislative session, a second funding source was initiated for FCN. Section 464.0198 was approved and established the Florida Center for Nursing Trust Fund. This fund permits the center to obtain voluntary contributions. Also approved in 2002 was an addendum to § 464.0195 that states:

> The Board of Nursing shall include on its initial and renewal application forms a question asking the nurse to voluntarily contribute to funding the Florida Center for Nursing in addition to paying the fees imposed at the time of licensure and licensure renewal. Revenues collected from nurses over and above the required fees shall be deposited in the Florida Center for Nursing Trust Fund and shall be used solely to support and maintain the goals and functions of the center.

As of March 31, 2004, 2,300 licensees have contributed $52,000. This represents an average contribution of $23 per individual. These funds have been used to sponsor a statewide conference on workforce issues, facilitate the drafting of a strategic plan to address the nursing shortage in Florida, and develop a tool for surveying nurses at the time of their license renewal. Without these funds, the FCN would not have been able to initiate these efforts.

Another important funding source is private foundations. The center's executive director has developed relationships across the state, identifying potential partners who share an interest in addressing the nursing shortage. Through this effort, a partnership has evolved with a foundation that identified the nursing shortage as one of its two priority areas for project funding. In 2004, the FCN and the foundation sought state funding that would be matched by the foundation and earmarked to establish demonstration projects to study nurse staffing and delivery models. The foundation successfully shepherded the proposal through the legislative session. As a result, the FCN has been designated to receive $250,000 from state funds that will be matched by the foundation. These funds will be used to conduct a three-year study of nurse staffing models in health care facilities in Florida. Clearly, this is a success story and an excellent example of a private-public partnership that is consistent with the mission of FCN and hopefully will improve the work environment for nurses and the quality of nursing care for Florida residents.

The Work of the FCN

As a part of its contract, the FCN must achieve certain deliverables. The board has established the vision, mission, and goals for the FCN as follows.

Vision

The Florida Center for Nursing is nationally recognized as the definitive source for information, trends, research, and forecasting about nurses and the dynamic nursing needs in Florida. The center is the focal point for creating synergistic partnerships and collaborative efforts among stakeholders in health care delivery.

Mission

- Address the issues of nursing supply and demand strategically to meet the needs of health care consumers in Florida.

- Generate and disseminate credible information to consumers of health care, professional organizations, health care providers, educational institutions, and legislators.
- Enhance and promote innovative recognition, reward, and renewal activities for nurses and potential nurses.

Goals

- The center for nursing will establish a research agenda to include data collection, analysis, and distribution.
- The center for nursing will publish a strategic plan to address issues of supply and demand to meet the needs of health care consumers in Florida.
- The center for nursing will describe a sustainability plan for its continuation.
- The center for nursing will design a strategy to address the image of nursing.
- The center for nursing will establish collaborative partnerships to facilitate the completion of its goals and objectives.
- The center for nursing will implement a communication plan for statewide sharing of information and resources.
- The center for nursing will formalize its structure and function to realize its mission and vision.

The FCN serves Florida and its nursing workforce; therefore, communication with the various constituencies is essential. By law, all FCN board meetings are open to the public. The board approves for distribution summary reports of meeting activities that are posted on the FCN Web-site. To save funds, stakeholder and constituency communication is electronic, and this approach appeals to younger, more technically savvy members. The FCN's Web-site, (http://www.FLCenterForNursing.org), has evolved into a valuable source of information. Electronic newsletters are sent quarterly to anyone submitting an e-mail address.

Accomplishments to Date

In its three years, the FCN has implemented a vigorous work program to meet its purposes and goals. By January 2004, the following activities have been initiated:

1. In cooperation with the Florida Board of Nursing, data are being collected for additional demographic information about

the Florida licensed nurse workforce. These data will be used to increase the public's knowledge about Florida nurses and to assist in long-range workforce planning.

2. Information-gathering events (stakeholder meetings) have been held in various regions of the state.

3. With Workforce Florida, Inc., the FCN cohosted a summit on nursing shortage, data, information, and strategy.

4. Staff and board members have published reports:
   - *Nursing Supply and Demand in Florida: Analysis of Nursing Licensure Data*
   - *Nursing Supply and Demand: Synthesis and Evaluation of Existing Florida Data*
   - *Florida Nursing Shortage,* a white paper of Florida-specific information from state and national sources
   - *Nursing Shortage Strategies: Effectiveness Evaluation Model*

5. Through collaboration with 12 professional organizations and state agencies, the FCN has wrote *Statewide Strategic Plan for Nursing Workforce in Florida.*

Lessons Learned

Building strong, positive relationships with state agencies (Board of Nursing, Department of Health, etc.) and professional groups is important to sustain funding and support for the center. If asked about the center, agency/professional representatives should have sufficient information to answer positively because any negative answers could result in concerted efforts to block the center's continuation. Both FCN staff and members of the board of directors have worked diligently to establish good relationships with legislators and state department representatives. In part, this is accomplished through information disseminated through the center's Web-site. In addition, the staff are committed to responding quickly to requests for assistance. In essence, a large part of the success in continuing funding is based on the image of the FCN.

Communication with all stakeholder groups is critical. The FCN board and staff have focused on the mission—a logical approach—and considered nursing the most important audience. With minimal staffing and resources, the work of the center was focused on data and compliance with required deliverables. In retrospect, there may have been value in identifying one or more projects that would have the potential to influence center funding, thus increasing resources. For the FCN, at least initially, that would have involved the Florida Legislature. Identifying a project significant valuable that the legislators would have read the report and used the results may have been a missed opportunity.

Sustainability is a continuing issue for FCN. As described previously, the center's base funding is a line item in the nonrecurring state budget, and the funding level is inadequate to meet statutory mandates. During the 2004 Florida legislative session, FNA proposed language that would enable the transfer of $5.00 per nurse license application and renewal to the Florida Board of Nursing Trust Fund to support the FCN. This funding stream would increase the annual budget allowance for the center to approximately $450,000 and would be ongoing. Support for the proposal was universal, and included members of the Board of Nursing, professional associations, state agencies, and elected officials. Thus, one could assume success would be ensured. Unfortunately, due to what was in essence a clerical error in the last hours of the legislative session, the provision (along with others) was omitted from the implementation bill. Investigation that uncovered the error also resulted in what seems to be a strong commitment to reintroduce the provision in 2005 and to track it more effectively.

To use a common business phrase, what is the bottom line? Being a state-mandated and funded-center has its challenges, but it also has opportunities. There is neutrality inherent in not being tied to either a private funding source or a professional association. To be successful, FCN must work from a broad perspective of nursing issues including all levels of practitioners and locations of employment. A part of the center's statutory mandate involves policy setting and gives an entry for influencing positive changes for nurses that will be beneficial to the residents of Florida. The challenge of positively influencing nursing workforce issues in the fourth largest state is daunting. Progress may not be as rapid as desired. This is in part related to funding levels. Nonetheless, the FCN exists and is moving forward with its work.

Although other stakeholder groups contribute to advocacy efforts to sustain funding for the FCN, the Florida Nurses Association (FNA) has provided the lion's share of these efforts. The positive relationships and consistent presence of FNA prior to and during legislative sessions have been essential. In addition, FCN staff have worked to keep legislators informed on the center's activities through electronic communications and distribution of updates to elected officials and their staff.

ARIZONA'S HEALTHCARE INSTITUTE (HCI)

Creation of the HCI

In contrast to state centers that focus solely on the nursing work-force, Arizona established the multiprofessional health care center. Created in 1996 by the Arizona Hospital and Healthcare Association (AzHHA), the Healthcare Institute (HCI) is the health care professions/workforce arm of the association. The AzHHA is the premier advocacy entity for over 80 hospitals and health care systems in the state. Two drivers led to the establishment of the institute: the chaotic restructuring efforts occurring within the state's hospitals and the constant swing between the supply of and demand for a variety of health care professions. The institute was created through $175,000 in seed funding contributed by the St. Luke's Charitable Health Trust (now St. Luke's Health Initiatives). The trust lent its support to the foundation of the institute because of its concern for the lack of coordinated, statewide efforts to address health care professions' issues and to create fundamental solutions to enduring, cyclical workforce problems. The mission of the HCI then and now is to respond to the health care needs of Arizonans through the development and support of a well-prepared, accessible workforce of qualified professionals and assistive personnel. The goals of the Institute include

- increasing communication and collaboration among health care professionals, educators, regulators, consumers, and employers
- collecting, analyzing, and publishing information relating to current and emerging health care workforce issues
- initiating studies and projects addressing the health care workforce needs of Arizonans and the demands of the state's health care systems.

Structure

The HCI advisory board, composed of a variety of representatives from many facets of the health care workforce, provides guidance and direction to the strategies and activities of the institute. The advisory board meets quarterly and, when necessary, convenes ad hoc committees, focused on specific programs and initiatives. The governing board of AzHHA is the authority to which the HCI reports and from which it receives both funding and strategic direction.

Funding

In 1996, to launch the HCI, St. Luke's Charitable Health Trust (SLCHT), a Phoenix-area conversion foundation, donated approximately $250,000 over a two-year period. These funds were designed to support infrastructure development. Salaries of the HCI staff were funded in part by AzHHA member dues and matching funds from SLCHT.

Concurrently, the HCI received a grant through the Robert Wood Johnson Foundation for the Colleagues in Caring project. AzHHA was able to match, dollar for dollar, the total amount committed by foundation. Matching funds consisted of contributions from hospitals, associations, foundations, and institutions of higher education. In 1999, the Colleagues in Caring grant, originally awarded for a three-year period, was renewed for a second three-year term, and matching funds were once again identified from similar sources of support.

In 2001, the HCI launched a major five-year initiative, the Campaign for Caring, focused on addressing the complex and substantive issues related to the state's shortage of health care professionals. A business plan and budget were developed and implemented in 2002 with a target fund-raising goal of $8 million over the five-year term of the campaign. To date, $5 million have been raised from a combination of hospitals and health care systems, Johnson & Johnson, and local foundations and philanthropic groups, including Arizona Blue Cross and Blue Shield.

Activities and Accomplishments to Date

All three HCI goals are reflected in its activities since its inception. Initial HCI activities were focused almost entirely on nursing because the emerging shortage would have such a profound impact on patient care. Subsequently, activities involving other shortage areas have been added. Nursing's activities, however, have served as the incubator for projects involving allied health.

Increasing Communication and Collaboration
- 1998: Created the day of dialogue model, which facilitated collaboration among various stakeholders and factions of specific health care professions. The first day of dialogue convened the physical therapy profession and resulted in a blueprint for action to improve access to physical therapy services in Arizona.

- 2000: Convened pharmacy day of dialogue.
- 2000: Began the discussion with nursing education leadership to explore increasing enrollment in Arizona's nursing education programs.
- 2002: Convened the medical technology profession in a day of dialogue with a focus on supporting the continuance of the University of Arizona's medical technology program.
- 2003: Convened the radiology/diagnostic imaging community in a day of dialogue.

Collecting and Analyzing Data

- 1996–present: Collected and disseminated data related to supply, preparation, and demands of health care professionals and workers. Data collection focused primarily on nurses, physical therapists, pharmacists, and laboratory and radiology personnel.
- 1999: Began preliminary conception of Arizona's response to forecasted shortage of nurses.

Quantitative and qualitative information and data collected through both the day of dialogue process and other methods have been used to direct policy-making decisions. Examples include the drafting of legislation to double the state's nursing education program enrollment capacity by 2007 and the creation of a new medical technician program at a community college.

Initializing Studies and Projects

- 1996–2002: Used funding from the Robert Wood Johnson Foundation for a nursing workforce study and project, Colleagues in Caring.
- 1996–2001: Provided initial leadership and funding for the Healing Community Project, an initiative that articulated Northern Arizona University's baccalaureate nursing program with multiple rural associate degree nursing programs in the state.
- 1996–2001: Led the development and implementation of a core curriculum model for the Maricopa Community Colleges Health Care Reform Commission, incorporating over 35 different health occupations programs in the core and across 10 different community colleges.
- 1998: Assumed responsibility for AzHHA's Salsbury Scholarship Program and directly linked the awarding of scholarships to students enrolled in programs with greatest demand.

- 1998: Assumed leadership role in quality and patient safety-related programs and services at AzHHA.
- 2000: Initiated work, including the development of a business plan, on Campaign for Caring, AzHHA's plan to address the state's nursing shortage.
- 2002: AzHHA sponsored and successfully lobbied for a bill to double the state's nursing school enrollment by 2007.

The impact of all these activities and efforts is evidenced by a 25% increase, to date, in nursing education program enrollment capacity and the presence of health care professions issues on repeated agendas of legislators, the governor, chambers of commerce, and the Arizona State Board of Regents.

Future Direction

In July 2002, the HCI updated its strategic plan to be more reflective of an integrated multidisciplinary approach to the delivery of health care to Arizonans. The HCI embraced the nine imperatives for enhancing the education practice, and regulation of health professionals outlined in *Understanding Change* (O'Neil, 2003b). These nine imperatives consist of questioning existing practice models, creating new partnerships, building consumer-oriented and accountable educational programs, increasing flexibility in work arrangements, realigning the image and practice of health work with the values of new workers, improving leadership at all levels, reconnecting health institutions and the communities they serve, deploying technology appropriately, and enhancing work environment.

The HCI's refocused strategic plan incorporates four imperatives-work environment, consumer-oriented and accountable education programs, leadership, and technology. In addition, the imperative of partnerships is integrated in all four initiatives, as can be seen in each of the following examples.

1. Enhance the health care work environment for increased patient and workforce satisfaction and safety.
- Partners: Arizona Organization of Nurse Executives (AzONE), Arizona Nurses Association (AzNA), and other professional associations
- Strategic activities:
  1. Sponsor forum—"What Patients Want, What Nurses Want, What Hospitals Want . . . And How to Get There."

   2. Monitor the public reporting of quality data projects.

   3. Continue to publish best practice guidelines through the patient safety task force.

   4. Monitor the work and progress of the commitment and passion workgroup of the Campaign for Caring, which focuses on this strategy.

2. Support the creation of consumer-oriented, practice-linked, and accountable health professions education programs.

- Partners: All health professions education programs in the state, AARP, health professions associations (AzNA, AzPA, etc.), presidents of community colleges, board of regents
- Strategic activities:
  1. Support the comprehensive implementation of bill 1260 (doubling nursing school enrollments).
  2. Monitor progress of Campaign for Caring education program grants aimed at enhancing the capacity of the state's nursing education programs.
  3. Sponsor an all-day summit aimed at understanding and integrating the cultures of health care and higher education.

3. Improve health care workforce leadership at all levels, from bedside to boardroom.

- Partners: Leadership of all health education programs in the state, AzONE, AzNA, other professional organizations
- Strategic activities:
  1. Convene a day of dialogue focused on this topic.
  2. Support the implementation of the AzNA's nursing leadership institute and consider as a model for other professional groups.

4. Anticipate and address the changes that will be brought to the health professions through biotechnology, genomics, and consumerism.

- Partners: All health professions education programs in the state, biotech and genomics leadership, lead consumer groups, including AARP
- Strategic activities:
  1. Become knowledgeable about all three movements as an advisory board.
  2. Sponsor a statewide summit on this topic.

Lesson Learned

While the new strategic plan does not change the direction of the HCI, it does require the refocusing of our attention from specific health care professions to more comprehensive health care workforce challenges. Through this refocusing, our efforts take on a more team-like orientation. A continual criticism of the health care workforce is its propensity for "splendid isolation" (O'Neil, 2003b) with each profession existing in its separate and distinct silo. Health care centers risk perpetuating the existence of these silos by studying each in isolation and isolated from the other groups and cultures impacting these professions. Nursing maintains a strong and pivotal role in the leadership of the HCI and incorporation of partners for its initiatives; however, we believe nurses and patients will benefit more from the integration rather than the isolation.

10

Next Steps

Brenda Cleary and Rebecca Rice

The final chapter in this journey toward taking the long view of nursing workforce issues is still being written. As we indicated earlier, almost all 50 states and the District of Columbia have embarked on this journey. Thirty states now have funded statewide entities addressing nursing workforce issues, and many other states have more loosely knit coalitions addressing this work. Two things we know for sure: Nursing is critical for the public's health, and nursing supply and demand concerns are not going away in the near future. Work must be done not only in the public sector but also in the private sector. Legislation can fund nursing education, provide scholarships, and influence some work environmental issues, such as mandatory overtime and staffing ratios. The very real work environmental concerns addressed in the Institute of Medicine's report (2004) must be addressed by the private sector. Nurses must play a pivotal role in this work, and nurses also must continue to refine data-collecting methods to make certain that all the stakeholders in nursing care have timely, objective information about the nursing workforce and its trends.

Many contributors shared their journeys in this book, and the subjects covered (nursing workforce entities, data, education, practice, recruitment, leadership, and policy) represent the wide gamut of concerns that are being addressed by nursing workforce entities around the country. Each of the examples in the chapters represented not the single work of one nursing leader effecting change in his or her sphere of influence; instead, all the examples derive their strength from the collective work of many leaders from different perspectives.

We believe firmly that this work cannot be accomplished in isolation. We are all better off for the shared wisdom of many in creating solutions to the problems we face as we attempt to make certain that our patients have sufficient numbers of nurses with the right education and experience to care for them.

Where are we going from here? We continue to meet annually. A second annual gathering of state nursing workforce initiatives was held in April 2004. We realize that much of our strength and many of our accomplishments are due to the generous, selfless sharing of best (and sometimes worst) practices with each other. Consequently, we are working collaboratively in organizing a communications network that will sustain our ability to share with one another. In other words, the best is yet to come.

References

Abrams, R. (2002, Jan. 28). Nursing woes: A turn in the troublesome road. *Healthleaders News*. Retrieved June 6, 2004 from http://www.healthleaders.com/news/feature1.php?contentid=31289

Aiken, L., Clarke, S., Cheung, R., Sloane, D., & Silber, J. (2003). Educational levels of hospital nurses and surgical patient mortality. *Journal of the American Medical Association, 290,* 1617–1624.

Aiken, L. H., Clarke, S. P., & Sloane, D. M. (2002). Hospital staffing, organization, and quality of care: Cross-national findings. *International Journal of Quality Health Care, 14*(1), 5–13.

Aiken, L. H., Clarke, S. P., Sloane, D. M., Sochalski, J., & Silber, J. H. (2002). Hospital nurse staffing and patient mortality, nurse burnout, and job dissatisfaction. *Journal of the American Medical Association, 288*(16), 1987–1993.

Aiken, L. H., Clarke, S. P., Sloane, D. M., Sochalski, J. A., Busse, R., Clarke, H., Giovannetti, P., Hunt, J., Rafferty, A. M., & Shamian, J. (2001). Nurses' reports on hospital care in five countries. *Health Affairs, 20*(3), 43–53.

Aiken, L., & Gwyther, M. (1995). Medicare funding of nurse education: The case for policy change. *Journal of the American Medical Association, 273,* 1528–1532.

Aiken, L. H., Havens, D. S., & Sloane, D. N. (2000). The magnet nursing services recognition program: A comparison of two groups of magnet hospitals. *American Journal of Nursing, 100*(3), 26–35.

Aiken, L., & Patrician, P. (2000). Measuring organizational traits of hospitals. The Revised Nursing Work Index. *Nursing Research, 49,* 146–153.

Aiken, L. H., & Sloane, D. M. (1997). Effects of organizational innovations in AIDS care on burnout among hospital nurses. *Work and Occupations, 24*(4), 455–479.

Aiken, L. H., Sloane, D. M., Lake, E. T., Sochalski, J., & Weber, A. L. (1999). Organization and outcomes of inpatient AIDS care. *Medical Care, 37*(8), 760–772.

Aiken, L. H., Smith, H. L., & Lake, E. T. (1994). Lower Medicare mortality among a set of hospitals known for good nursing care. *Medical Care, 32*(8), 771–787.

American Association of Colleges of Nursing. (2003). *AACN's nursing faculty shortage fact sheet.* Washington, DC: Author.

American Association of Colleges of Nursing. (2004a). *AACN's 23rd annual survey of institutions with baccalaureate and higher degree nursing programs.* Washington, DC: Author.

American Association of Colleges of Nursing. (2004b). *Nursing faculty shortage facts and factors.* Washington, DC: Author.

American Association of Colleges of Nursing. (2004c). *Thousands of students turned away from the nation's nursing schools despite sharp increase in enrollment.* Washington, DC: Author.

American Association of Colleges of Nursing. (2004d). *2003–2004 Enrollment and graduations in baccalaureate and graduate programs in nursing.* Washington, DC: Author.

American Association of Colleges of Nursing/American Organization of Nurse Executives. (1995). *A model for differentiated nursing practice.* Supported by a grant from the Robert Wood Johnson Foundation.

American Hospital Association. (1983). *The National Commission on Nursing: Summary report and recommendations.* Chicago: Author.

American Hospital Association. (2002). *How hospitals can build a thriving workforce.* Chicago: Author.

American Nurses Association. (1995). *Scope and standards for nurse administrators.* Washington, DC: American Nurses Publishing.

American Nurses Association. (2002). *A call to the nation.* Washington, DC: American Nurses Association.

American Organization of Nurse Executives. (January, 2000). *Nurse recruitment and retention study.* Chicago: Author.

Arizona Hospital and Healthcare Association. Retrieved February 10, 2004, from http://www.azhha.org

Baggs, J. G., Schmitt, M. H., Mushlin, A. I., Eldredge, D. H., Oakes, D., & Hutson, A. D. (1997). Nurse-physician collaboration and satisfaction with the decision-making process in three critical care units. *American Journal of Critical Care, 6*(5), 393–399.

Bednash, G. (2000). The decreasing supply of registered nurses: Inevitable future or call to action. *Journal of the American Medical Association, 283*(22), 2985–2987.

Benner, P. (1984). *From novice to expert: Excellence and power in clinical nursing practice.* Menlo Park, CA: Addison-Wesley.

Benner, P. A., Tanner, C. A., & Chesla, C. A. (1996). *Expertise in nursing practice: Caring, clinical judgment, and ethics.* New York: Springer.

Blegen, M. A. (1993). Nurses job satisfaction: A meta-analysis of related variables. *Nursing Research, 42*(1), 36–41.

Bleich, M. R. (2003). Managing, leading, and following. In P. Yoder-Wise (Ed.), *Leading and managing in nursing* (3rd ed.). St. Louis: Mosby.

Bleich, M. R., Hewlett, P. O., Santos, S. R., Rice, R. B., Cox, K. S., & Richmeier, S. (2003). Analysis of the nursing workforce crisis: A call to action. *American Journal of Nursing, 103*(4), 66–74.

Boland, D., & Carlisle, P. (2003). Impact of the Nursing 2000 model. In L. Briggs, S. E. Merck, & B. Mitchell, *Collaboration for the promotion of nursing.* Indianapolis, IN: Sigma Theta Tau International.

Boyle, D. K., Bott, M. J., Hansen, H. E., Woods, C. Q., & Taunton, R. L. (1999). Managers' leadership and critical care nurses' intent to stay. *American Journal of Critical Care, 8*(6), 361–371.

Briggs, L., Merk, S. E., & Mitchell, B. (2003). *Collaboration for the promotion of nursing.* Indianapolis, IN: Sigma Theta Tau International.

Brown, B. (2002, April 8). Chart a course: Survey reveals nursing dissatisfactions—Now, it's time to act for change. *NurseWeek.* Retrieved April 15, 2004, from http://www.nurseweek.com/ednote/02/040802b_print.html

Brunell, M. L., & Rice, R. (2003). *State nursing workforce center survey results.* Unpublished manuscript.

Buerhaus, P. I. (1999). Is a nursing shortage on the way? *Nursing Management, 30*(2), 54–55.

Buerhaus, P. I., Staiger, D. O., & Auerbach, D. I. (2000). Implications of an aging registered nurse workforce. *Journal of the American Medical Association, 283*(22), 2948–2954.

California State University. (1998, September). *Education bond makes ballot as 1997–1998 legislative session concludes.* Retrieved June 6, 2004, from http://www.calstate.edu/GA/LegReport/leg090498.shtml

Cassard, S. D., Weisman, D. J., Gordon, D. L., & Wong, R. (1994). The impact of unit-based self-management by nurses on patient outcomes. *Health Services Research, 29*(4), 415–433.

Cleary, B. L., Lacey, L. M., & Beck-Warden, M. (1998). Estimating the market for nursing personnel in North Carolina. *Image: Journal of Nursing Scholarship, 30,* 335–338.

Cohen, S., & Sherrod, D. (2003). *Surviving the nursing shortage: Strategies for recruitment and retention.* Marblehead, MA: Opus Communications.

Corey-Lisle, P., Tarzian, A. J., Cohen, M. Z., & Trinkoff, A. M. (1999). Healthcare reform. Its effects on nurses. *Journal of Nursing Administration, 29*(3), 30–37.

Davidson, H., Folcarelli, P. H., Crawford, S., Duprat, L. J., & Clifford, J. C. (1997). The effects of health care reforms on job satisfaction and voluntary turnover among hospital-based nurses. *Medical Care, 35*(6), 634–645.

Department of Health and Human Services, Centers for Disease Control and Prevention, National Center for Health Statistics. (2004). *Summary measures of population health: Report of findings on methodological and data issues.* DHHS publication number (PHS) 2004–1258.

Ehrmann, S. (1999). Access and/or quality? Redefining choices in the third revolution. *Educom Review, 34*(5), 1–8.

Eisenberg, J. M., Bowman, C. C., & Foster, N. E. (2001). Does a healthy health care workplace produce higher-quality care? *The Joint Commission Journal on Quality Improvement, 27*(9), 444–457.

Elsass, P. M., & Veiga, J. F. (1997). Job control and job strain: A test of three models. *Journal of Occupational Health Psychology, 2*(3), 195–211.

Fagin, C. (1999, March 16). Where are the nurses? *New York Times,* p. F7.

Fagin, C. (2000). *Essays on nursing leadership.* New York: Springer Publishing.

Ferguson, E. (1983). Preface. In M. L. McClure, M. A. Poulin, M. D. Sovie, & M. A. Wandelt (Eds.), *Magnet hospitals: Attraction and retention of professional nurses.* Kansas City, MO: The American Academy of Nursing, vii.

Ferguson, V. (1990). Preface. *Nursing Clinics of North America, 25*(3), xiii.

FitchRatings. (2003, May). *Nursing shortage update.* Retrieved May 1, 2004, from http://www.fitchratings.com/corporate/reports/report.cfm?rpt_id=172154

Florida Center for Nursing. (2001). § 464.0195. Retrieved April 1, 2004, from http://election.dos.state.fl.us/laws/02laws/ch_2002-229.pdf

Flower, J. (1995). Collaboration: The new leadership. *Health Forum Journal, 28*(6), 20–25.

Foley, B. J., Kee, C. C., Minick, P., Harvey, S. S., & Jennings, B. M. (2002). Characteristics of nurses and nurses and hospital work environments that foster satisfaction and clinical expertise. *Journal of Nursing Administration, 32*(5), 273–282.

Gardner, D. B. (1998). *Effects of conflict types and power style use among health professionals in interdisciplinary team collaboration.* Unpublished doctoral dissertation, George Mason University, Fairfax, VA.

Grantmakers in Health. (2003). *A profile of new health foundations.* Retrieved June 14, 2004, from http://www.gih.org/usr_doc/2003_Profile_Report.pdf

Havens, D. S. (2001). Comparing nursing infrastructure and outcomes: ANCC magnet and nonmagnet CNEs report. *Nursing economics, 19*(6), 258–266.

Havens, D. S., & Aiken, L. H. (1999). Shaping systems to promote desired outcomes: The magnet hospital model. *Journal of Nursing Administration, 29*(2), 14–20.

Health Care Advisory Board. (2000a, January 27). *Job characteristics, not career prospects, drive nurse retention.* Washington, DC: Author.

Health Care Advisory Board. (2000b). *Reversing the flight of talent: Executive briefing.* Washington, DC: Author:

Helgesen, S. (1995). *The web of inclusion.* New York: Doubleday.

Hemsley-Brown, J., & Foskett, N. (1999). Career desirability: Young people's perception of nursing as a career. *Journal of Advanced Nursing, 29*(6), 1342–1349.

Hinshaw, A. S. (2002). Building magnetism into health organizations. In M. McClure & A. S. Hinshaw (Eds.), *Magnet hospitals revisited.* Washington, D.C.: American Nurses Publishing.

Hinshaw, A. S., Smeltzer, C. H., & Atwood, J. R. (1987). Innovative retention strategies for nursing staff. *Journal of Nursing Administration, 17*(6), 8–16.

Institute of Medicine. (1983). *Nursing and nursing education: Public policies and private actions.* Washington, DC: National Academy Press.

Institute of Medicine. (2000). *To err is human: Building a safer health system.* Washington, DC: National Academy Press.

Institute of Medicine. (2001). *Crossing the quality chasm: A new health system for the 21st century.* Washington, DC: National Academy Press.

Institute of Medicine. (2003). *Health professions education: A bridge to quality.* Washington, DC: National Academy Press.

Institute of Medicine, Committee on the Work Environment for Nurses and Patient Safety. (2004). *Keeping patients safe: Transforming the work environment of nurses.* Washington, DC: National Academy Press.

Jacox, A. K. (1982). Role restructuring in hospital nursing. In L.

Aiken & S. Gortner (Eds.), *Nursing in the 1980s—crises, opportunities, challenges* (pp. 75–99). Philadelphia: Lippincott.

Jones, C. B. (1990a). Staff nurse turnover costs: Part I, a conceptual model. *Journal of Nursing Administration, 20*(4), 18–22.

Jones, C. B. (1990b). Staff nurse turnover costs: Part II, measurement and results. *Journal of Nursing Administration, 20*(5), 27–32.

Jones, C. B. (1996). Registered nurse turnover and the changing health care system. *Nursingconnections, 9*(1), 35–48.

Kalding, T. H., Vermont Organization of Nurse Leaders, and Vermont Association of Hospitals and Health Systems (retrieved Nov. 22, 2003). *Report on nursing in Vermont.* Montpelier, VT: Author.

Kalliath, T. J., & Beck, A. (2001). Is the path to burnout and turnover paved by a lack of supervisory support? A structural equations test. *New Zealand Journal of Psychology, 30*(2), 72–80.

Karasek, R., & Theorell, T. (1990). *Healthy work, stress, productivity, and reconstruction of working life.* New York: Basic Books.

Keating, S., & Sechrist, K. (2001, January 31). The nursing shortage in California: The public policy role of the California Strategic Planning Committee for Nursing. *Online Journal of Issues in Nursing, 6*(1). Retrieved 11/20/04 from http://www.nursingworld.org/ojin/topic14/tpc14_2.htm

Kimball, B., & O'Neil, E. (2001). *Healthcare's human crisis: The American nursing shortage.* Princeton, NJ: The Robert Wood Johnson Foundation.

Kinnaman, M. L. (1999). *A concept analysis of interdisciplinary collaboration* (Unpublished manuscript). Kansas City: University of Missouri–Kansas City.

Kinnaman, M. L., & Bleich, M. R. (2004). Collaboration: Aligning resources to create and sustain partnerships. *Journal of Professional Nursing, 20*(5), 310–322.

Knaus, W. A., Draper, E. A., Wagner, D. P., & Zimmerman, J. E. (1986). An evaluation of outcome from intensive care in major medical centers. *Annals of Internal Medicine, 104*(3), 410–418.

Langemo, D. K., Anderson, J., & Volden, C. M. (2002). Nursing quality outcome indicators: The North Dakota study. *Journal of Nursing Administration, 32*(2), 98–105.

Laschinger, H. S., & Havens, D. S. (1996a). Staff nurse empowerment and perceived control over nursing practice. *Journal of Nursing Administration, 26*(9), 27–35.

Laschinger, H. S., & Havens, D. S. (1996b). Testing Kanter's theory: Staff RN perceptions of work empowerment, control over nursing practice, satisfaction and work effectiveness. *Journal of Nursing Administration, 26*(9), 27–35.

Laschinger, H. S., & Havens, D. S. (1997). The effect of workplace empowerment and perceptions of occupational mental health and work effectiveness. *Journal of Nursing Administration, 27*(6), 42–50.

Laschinger, H. S., Shamian, J., & Thomson, D. (2001). Impact of magnet hospital characteristics on nurses: Perceptions of trust, burnout, quality of care, and work satisfaction. *Nursing Economics, 19*(5), 209–219.

Lenburg, C. (1999, September). The framework, concepts and methods of the competency outcomes and performance assessment (COPA) model. *Online Journal of Issues in Nursing.* Retrieved April 1, 2004, from http://nursingworld.org/ojin/topic10/tpc10_2.htm

Leveck, M. L., & Jones, C. B. (1996). The nursing practice environment, staff retention, and quality of care. *Research in Nursing and Health, 19,* 331–343.

Longest, B. (2002). *Health policymaking in the United States* (3rd ed.). Chicago: Health Administration Press.

Lucas, M. D., Atwood, J. R., & Hagaman, R. (1993). Replication and validation of anticipated turnover model for urban registered nurses. *Nursing Research, 42*(1), 29–35.

Malloch, K., Davenport, S., & Hatler, C. (2003). Using benchmarking for planning and outcomes monitoring. *Journal of Nursing Administration, 33*(10), 538–543.

Mark, B., Salyer, J., & Wan, T. T. H. (2003). Professional nursing practice: Impact on organizational and patient outcomes. *Journal of Nursing Administration, 33*(4), 224–234.

Maryland Commission on the Crisis in Nursing. (2001, January). *Interim report to the governor and the state legislature.* Annapolis: Author.

McClure, M. L., & Hinshaw, A. S. (2002). *Magnet hospitals revisited: Attraction and retention of professional nurses.* Washington, DC: American Nurses Publishing.

McClure, M. L., Poulin, M. A., Sovie, M. D., & Wandelt, M. A. (1983). *Magnet hospitals: Attraction and retention of professional nurses.* Kansas City, MO: American Academy of Nursing.

Mercer, W. M. (1999, August). *Attracting and retaining registered nurses—Survey results.* Chicago: Author.

Mississippi Board of Nursing. (2003). *Annual report.* Retrieved June 14, 2004, from http://www.msbn.state.ms.us/pdf/anreport03.pdf

Mitchell, P. H., Armstrong, S., Simpson, T. F., & Lentz, M. (1989). American Association of Critical-Care Nurses demonstration project: Profile of excellence in critical care nursing. *Heart Lung, 18*(3), 219–237.

Moore, G. (2002). *Crossing the chasm.* New York: Harper Collins.

National Council of State Boards of Nursing. (2004). *Values.* Retrieved June 14, 2004, from http://www.ncsbn.org/about/index.asp

National League for Nursing. (2003). *Annual survey of schools of nursing.* New York: Author.

Needleman, J., Buerhaus, P., Mattke, S., Stewart, M., & Zelevinsky, K. (2002). Nurse-staffing levels and the quality of care in hospitals. *New England Journal of Medicine, 346*(22), 1715–1722.

North Carolina Center for Nursing. Retrieved February 10, 2004, from http://www.nurseNC.org

Nursing Executive Center (2000). *Reversing the flight of talent.* Volume I. Washington, DC: The Advisory Board Company.

Nursing 2000. (2002). *Annual report.* Indianapolis, IN: Author.

Nursing 2000. (2003). *Annual report.* Indianapolis, IN: Author.

Nursing Workforce Planning Group. (2001). *A call to action: VA's response to the national nursing shortage.* Washington, DC: Department of Veterans' Affairs, Veterans Health Administration.

O'Neil, E. (2003a, January). *Centering on change.* Retrieved April 14, 2004, from http://www.futurehealth.ucsf.edu/from_the_director_0103.html

O'Neil, E. (2003b). *Understanding change.* Retrieved April 14, 2004, from http://www. futurehealth.ucsf.edu/from_the_director_0103.html

O'Neil, E. (2004). *Centering on . . . teamwork in health care.* Retrieved March 2004 from http://futurehealth.ucsf.edu/from_the_director_0204.html

O'Neil, E., & Coffman, J. (1998). *Strategies for the future of nursing: Changing roles, responsibilities, and employment for registered nurses.* San Francisco: Jossey Bass.

Osipow, S. H., & Spokane, A. R. (1981). *Occupational stress inventory manual.* Lutz, FL: Psychological Assessment Resources, Inc.

Peter, D. Hart Research Associates. (2001, April). *The nurse shortage: Perspectives from current direct care nurses and former direct care nurses.* Washington, DC: The Federation of Nurses and Health Professionals.

Peters, T. (2002). Foreword. In B. Clarke & R. Crossland (Eds.), *The leaders' voice* (p. ix). New York: Select Books.

Pew Health Professions Commission. (1995). *Critical challenges: Revitalizing the health professions for the twenty-first century.*

Retrieved May 6, 2004, from http://futurehealth.ucsf.edu/ pdf_files/challenges.pdf

Polit, D., & Hungler, B. (1977). *Essentials of nursing research: Methods, appraisal, and utilization.* Philadelphia: Lippincott Raven.

Porter, R. W., & Prysor-Jones, S. (1997). *Making a difference in policy and programs: A guide for researchers.* Washington, DC: U.S. Agency for International Development, Africa Bureau, Office of Sustainable Development.

Prescott, P. (2000). The enigmatic nursing workforce. *Journal of Nursing Administration, 30*(2), 59–65.

Price, J. L., & Mueller, C. W. (1981). A causal model of turnover for nurses. *Academy of Management Journal, 24*(3), 543–565.

Robert Wood Johnson Executive Nurse Fellows Program. Retrieved February 10, 2004, from http://www.futurehealth.ucsf.edu

Robinson, J. E. (2003). Providing leadership in rural health care: The evolving role of virtual teams in managing projects. *Patient Care Management, 19*(1), 2–4.

Sainfort, F., Karsh, B., Booske, B., & Smith, M. (2001). Applying quality improvement principles to achieve healthy work environments. *Journal of Quality Improvement, 27*(9), 469–483.

Santos, S. R., Carroll, C. A., Cox, K. S., Teasley, S. L., Simon, S. D., Bainbridge, L., Cunningham, M., & Ott, L. (2003). Baby boomer nurses bearing the burden of care: A four-site study of stress, strain, and coping for inpatient registered nurses. *Journal of Nursing Administration, 33*(4), 243–250.

Santos, S. R., & Cox, K. (2000). Workplace adjustment and intergenerational differences between matures, baby boomers, and generation Xers. *Nursing Economics, 18*(1), 7–13.

Schmid, L., & Lacey, L. (2000). *Using the nursing supply model to estimate the future supply of registered nurses: A test and critique.* Retrieved April 15, 2004, from http://www.nursenc. org/research/NSMpaper.pdf

Seago, J. A., Ash, M., Spetz, J., Coffman, J., & Grumbach, K. (2001). Hospital registered nurse shortages: Environmental, patient, and institutional predictors. *Health Services Research, 36*(5), 831–852.

Sechrist, K. R., & Lewis E. M. (1996). *Planning for California's nursing work force: Final report of the nursing work force and education forecasting initiative, California Strategic Planning Committee for Nursing.* Sacramento, CA: ONE-California.

Sechrist K. R., Lewis, E. M., & Rutledge, D. N. (1999). *Planning for California's nursing work force: Phase II final report, California*

Strategic Planning Committee for Nursing. Sacramento, CA: Association of California Nurse Leaders. Retrieved April 15, 2004, from http://www.ucihs.uci.edu/cspcn

Sechrist, K. R., Lewis, E. M., Rutledge, D. N., & Keating, S. B. (2002). *Planning for California's nursing work force: Phase III final report, California Strategic Planning Committee for Nursing.* Sacramento, CA: Association of California Nurse Leaders. Retrieved April 15, 2004, from http://www.ucihs.uci.edu/cspcn

Southern Regional Education Board. (2002, February). *SREB study indicates serious shortage of nursing faculty.* Atlanta, GA: Author.

Staiger, D., Auerbach, D., & Buerhaus, P. (2000). Expanding career opportunities for women and the declining interest in nursing as a career. *Nursing Economic$, 18*(5), 230–236.

State of California, Employment Development Department, Labor Market Information. (1998, July). *Employment projections by occupation.* Sacramento, CA : Author.

Sullivan, E. (2003). *Becoming influential: A guide for nurses.* Saddle River, NJ: Princeton Hall.

Taunton, R. L., Boyle, D. K., Woods, C. Q., Hansen, H. E., & Bott, M. J. (1997). Manager leadership and retention of hospital staff nurses. *Western Journal of Nursing Research, 19*(2), 205–226.

U.S. Bureau of Labor Statistics. (1998). *1998–99 Occupational outlook handbook.* Washington, DC: U.S. Department of Labor, 1998.

U.S. Bureau of Labor Statistics. (2002). *A century of change: The U.S. labor force, 1950–2050.* Retrieved February 15, 2004, from http://www.bls.gov/opub/mlr/2002/05/art2full.pdf

U.S. Bureau of Labor Statistics (2004, February 11). *BLS releases 2002–2012 employment projections.* Retrieved April 1, 2004, from http://www.bls.gov/emp

U.S. Department of Health and Human Services. (1988). *The secretary's commission on nursing, Volumes I and II.* Washington, DC: Author.

U.S. Department of Health and Human Services, Bureau of Health Professions, Division of Nursing, National Advisory Council on Nursing Education and Practice. (1995). *Report on the basic registered nurse workforce, 1995.* Retrieved February 4, 2004, from http://bhpr.hrsa.gov/nursing/nacnep/workforce.htm

U.S. Department of Health and Human Services, Bureau of Health Professions, Division of Nursing. (2002, February). *National sample survey of registered nurses.* Washington, DC: Author.

U.S. Department of Health and Human Services, Centers for Disease Control and Prevention, National Center for Health Statistics. (2004). *Summary measures of population health: Report of findings on methodological and data issues.* DHHS Publication number (PHS) 2004-1258.

U.S. Department of Health and Human Services, Health Resources and Services Administration, Bureau of Health Professions, National Center for Health Workforce Analysis. (2002). *Projected supply, demand, and shortages of registered nurses, 2000–2020.* Retrieved May 10, 2004, from ftp://ftp.hrsa.gov/bhpr/national-center/rnproject.pdf

U.S. Department of Labor. (2004). *Local solutions with national applications to address health care industry labor shortages.* Retrieved April 1, 2004, from http://www.doleta.gov/BRG/IndProf/Health.cfm

U.S. Government Accounting Office. (2001, July). *Nursing workforce: Emerging nurse shortages due to multiple factors.* (No. GAO-01-944). Washington, DC: Author.

Veteran's Administration Health Care Amendments of 1980, Public Law 96-330 Pilot Program and Study, 96th Congress, Washington, DC. (1980).

Veteran's Administration Call to Action and Veterans Administration National Nursing Workforce Planning Group (2001).

Wakefield, M. (2003). Health care policy or politics: Which prevails in 2003? *Nursing Economics$, 21*(1), 47–48.

Weiss, C. (1977). Research for policy's sake: The enlightenment function of social research. *Policy Analysis, 3*(4), 531–545.

Wild, L. R., & Mitchell, P. H. (2000). Quality pain management outcomes: The power of place. *Outcomes Management for Nursing Practice, 4*(3), 136–143.

Wilson, C. S., & Mitchell, B. S. (1999). Nursing 2000: Collaboration to promote careers in registered nursing. *Nursing Outlook, 47*(2), 56–61.

Workforce Investment Act of 1998. PL 105-220, 1998 HR 1385. Retrieved June 15, 2004, from http://www.usdoj.gov/crt/508/508law.html

Zemke, R., Raines, C., & Filipczak, B. (2000). *Generations at work: Managing the Clash of veterans, boomers, Xers, and nexters in your workplace.* New York: AMACOM.

Appendix A

Colleagues in Caring Minimum Supply-Side Data Elements

During the Colleagues in Caring program sponsored by the Robert Wood Johnson Foundation, participating state centers collaborated to define the structure of a standard data set that could be used by states to measure and profile their nursing workforce. The result was a minimum data set of 13 questions and 33 data fields, each considered essential to successful workforce planning.

The answer categories used in each question are the recommended minimum. If additional categories are desired or needed in a particular state to address policy issues, the categories can be expanded. (Be sure, however, that any expanded categories can be aggregated back into the original groups so that longitudinal and cross-state comparisons can be made.) The inclusion of Social Security number may be problematic in some states, and may result in lower survey return rates. It is not a mandatory field, but some other unique identifier (such as nursing license number) is a necessity if you intend to track the work patterns of individuals over time.

If this series of questions is to be used for both RNs and LPNs in a state, there should be an additional item included that allows researchers to know which RNs are also actively licensed as LPNs in that state so that double counting can be avoided. Also, some items may need to be adjusted to better fit the LPN workforce (e.g., remove the question about advanced practice education, include the LPN education program type in the education listing, etc.).

PERSONAL DEMOGRAPHICS

Check **all** *educational programs completed* and fill in the *year graduated* from each.

Check	Type of program	Year graduated
☐	diploma in nursing	_ _ _ _
☐	associate degree, nursing	_ _ _ _
☐	associate degree, other field	_ _ _ _
☐	baccalaureate degree, nursing	_ _ _ _
☐	baccalaureate degree, other	_ _ _ _
☐	master's degree, nursing	_ _ _ _
☐	master's degree, other	_ _ _ _
☐	doctoral degree, nursing	_ _ _ _
☐	doctoral degree, other	_ _ _ _

Check **all** advanced practice educational programs completed.

- ☐ nurse practitioner (NP)
- ☐ clinical nurse specialist (CNS)
- ☐ certified nurse midwife (CNM)
- ☐ certified nurse anesthetist (CRNA)

In what year were you born?

To which racial/ethnic group do you belong? (Check only one.)

- ☐ White, not of Hispanic origin
- ☐ Black, not of Hispanic origin
- ☐ Hispanic
- ☐ American Indian/Alaskan native
- ☐ Asian/Pacific islander
- ☐ Other racial group
- ☐ Multiracial

Indicate your gender (Check only one.)   ☐ Male   ☐ Female

What is the Zip code for your current home address?

_____

What is your Social Security number?

_____

Alternate:

What is your RN license number?

_____

EMPLOYMENT STATUS

Check the box that describes your current nursing employment status. (Employment in nursing means **any** job that requires you to hold an active license to practice as a nurse—not just staff nurse or direct care positions.) (Check only **one** box.)

- ☐ actively employed in a paid position in nursing
- ☐ working in nursing but ONLY as a volunteer
- ☐ actively working in a paid position in health care but not in nursing
- ☐ actively working, but not in nursing or in health care
- ☐ unemployed and seeking work as a nurse
- ☐ temporarily inactive as a nurse
- ☐ retired from nursing or permanently inactive as a nurse

If you are actively working in nursing, whether paid or as a volunteer, please continue to the next item. If you checked any of the other options, please stop here.

If you work in more than one nursing position, please answer each of the following questions as it pertains to your *primary* position—the one where you spend the most time each month.

Does your primary nursing position involve providing direct care services to patients/families?

- ☐ yes   ☐ no

How many hours did you work last week in your primary nursing position? _____

(Do not count on-call hours. Do count vacation or sick-leave hours if they were paid.)

Check *one setting* that best describes where you practice in your primary nursing position.

☐ hospital   ☐ long-term care
☐ ambulatory care   ☐ home health care
☐ public/community health   ☐ nursing education
☐ occupational health   ☐ school health
☐ insurance company   ☐ other setting

Check *one position title* that best describes your primary nursing position.

☐ staff nurse/general duty nurse
☐ quality assurance, infection control
☐ discharge planner, case manager
☐ utilization review, outcomes management, other insurance-related role
☐ educator (school or inservice education)
☐ researcher, consultant
☐ nurse practitioner, certified nurse midwife, clinical nurse specialist, nurse anesthetist
☐ facility or nursing department administrator/supervisor/manager
☐ team leader/charge nurse/shift manger/head nurse
☐ other

What is the Zip code of your primary practice location?

_____

(If you deliver care in multiple locations, such as home care, give the Zip code of your home office.)

The following two questions are recommended in addition to those identified in the CIC Minimum Supply Data Set. These two questions will help states obtain more accurate counts of their workforce now that the Multi-State Licensure Compact is in force.

Please *list all states* in which you hold an *active license* as an RN:

_____

Please *list all states* in which you are *currently practicing*.

_____

Index